CLINICAL APPROACH TO Headache

DR. C.P. MALL

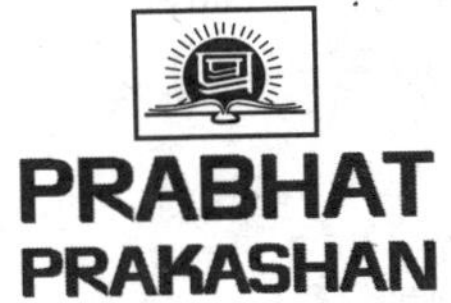

PRABHAT PRAKASHAN

Published by
PRABHAT PRAKASHAN PVT. LTD.
4/19 Asaf Ali Road,
New Delhi-110002 (INDIA)
e-mail: prabhatbooks@gmail.com

ISBN 978-93-5488-665-2
CLINICAL APPROACH TO HEADACHE
by Dr. C.P. Mall

Edition
First, 2023

Price
₹ 250 (Rupees Two Hundred Fifty Only)

Printed at
Japan Art, Delhi

Author's Note

"HEADACHE" is a very common problem and almost every doctor whether he be a physician or neurologist or psychiatrist or general practitioner daily see lots of patients of headache. However, "Headache" as a symptom has not been studied much. Little attention is being paid on this subject in under graduate-teaching. As a result, very few doctors are able to understand the real mechanism and patterns of headache and how to treat them.

As very few books are available on this subject, a practical guide was needed so as to explore a clearer understanding about headache. Therefore, this book aims to shed light on the factors that could be the cause for this common symptom that afflicts many people.

Most of the books available in the market are usually exhaustive and theoretical. This book is presented as a handy and practical guide for medical students and practitioners. It aims to be informative and useful to the patients and their care givers as well. The book has been written in an easy to understandable manner.

A practical approach towards cases of headache can begin by focusing on how to record a proper history by asking the patients to maintain a headache diary, giving importance for a better relation and communication between the doctor and the patient. Thereby, developing the skill to differentiate different types of headache and arriving at the correct diagnosis. Practical tips like a list of alarming signs have been given to know when to be alarmed and undergo for expensive investigations like CT or MRI to rule out serious medical conditions.

A holistic approach of management including pharmacological and non-pharmacological methods along with importance of maintaining balanced and stress-free lifestyle has been emphasized.

The book is unique in the sense that it is based on clinical ground. The book begins with Chapter with "Introduction" to the topic. In the next chapter, a brief "History of Headache" is described. The third chapter presents "Causes and Triggers of Headache" and the fourth chapter is about "Certain facts about Headache" which enables the reader to have a better understanding about the features of different types of headache.

The fifth chapter is on "When is Headache serious enough to seek medical help". It is very important as it highlights some important facts about headache and describes alarming symptoms which enables the clinicians to be alert and take prompt measures to make correct diagnosis and start treatment as early as possible.

Similarly, the chapter on migraine describes not only clinical details about it but also points out the relation and effect of migraine in special situations like menstruation, pregnancy, breast feeding, stroke and obesity. Effects of overuse of medication has been discussed in the chapter on "Chronic Migraine". "Migraine in association with other Non-Headache illnesses" has been described in a separate chapter.

In the chapter on "Treatment of Migraine" treatment of both acute migraine and prevention of migraine has been illustrated with name of commonly used medicines and its doses. Even non-pharmacological treatment has also been mentioned for a broader understanding about the better management of migraine patients. A list of suggestion to migraine patients have also been given at the end of this chapter.

The chapter on "Tension Type Headache" and "Cluster Headache" have been described in such a way that it makes concept clear regarding both types of headache and its management. "Secondary Headache" with some common causes has been also discussed in a separate chapter. The final chapter deals with "Management and Treatment of Headache" which is unique in the sense that it addresses importance of maintaining a headache calendar and proper communication between the doctor and the patient along with importance of balanced outlook in life and maintaining regular daily routine.

While most books on "Headache" by successful competitors are descriptive in nature, this book is more towards a practical understanding and approach to a case of headache. It is based on clinical grounds and is written in easy to understand manner and focuses on how to differentiate between different types of headaches. It also targets to enlighten the reader's understanding about when to go for expensive investigations like CT or MRI of the brain as it is very important in cases of secondary headache while patients of primary headache don't require it.

This book can serve as a practical guide to medical students and practitioners. It aims to clear the concepts about headache, enables the readers to understand all about what is known about headache and how to make a correct diagnosis as it focuses on the importance of detailed history taking, maintaining a headache calendar and proper physical and mental status examination. After going through the book, the clinician will be able to determine when the headache of the patient is serious and hence needs to be investigated and properly treated. The book describes about both pharmacological as well as non-pharmacological methods of management. Thus, it throws light on holistic approach in managing the patient. This is a novel approach and it gives practical tips to the readers.

I hope this book will be helpful to the readers by gaining a better understanding of what is known and what is not known about headache allowing them to explore diagnosis, treat and manage the patients in a better way with this knowledge in hand.

Acknowledgements

After I completedmy M.D in Psychiatry in the year 1992 from King George's Medical College, Lucknow. I joined government service in Uttar Pradesh where I got opportunity to work in both general hospitals from primary health centers to district hospitals as well as in specialized psychiatric centers like Mental Hospital in different capacities ranging from medical officer, senior consultant (psychiatrist) to Director & Superintendent-in-chief, where I came across many patients suffering from different types of headaches which made their life measurable. I developed special interest in this subject and gained experience from which grew the understanding of headaches. I felt that despite it being very common problem, there is lack of awareness and understanding even among medical practitioners. This prompted me to write this book on "Clinical Approach to Headache". I went through the available literature on it which enlightened my knowledge. I will like to thank all those authors who have contributed in this field.

Writing a book is not an easy job. It requires lot of patience and labour. It took me years to compile the information I have gathered over the course of my experience and reading. In this journey I have been fortunate to get assistance and help from my computer expert Shri Garvit Gulati without whom this book could not have seen light of the day. I have no words to thank and appreciate him for his selfless, sincere services rendered to me.

My family specially my children, Tanmay and Tanvika have been very supportive and encouraged me to write this book. I am thankful to my parents and teachers who mentored me in such a way that I could accomplish this task.

I am indebted to my patients who taught me about headaches and enabled me to clear my concepts about it and motivated me to write this book.

I dedicate my book "Clinical Approach to Headache" to my parents, teachers, family, friends and all my patients.

Contents

1
CHAPTER

Introduction

Headache is one of the most common complaints which disturb us. It ranges from mild, infrequent, negligible to severe, almost decapitating one. Most of the time it is ignored but at times it produces lot of problem and one is so disturbed that he has to take rest and may even be unable to do any work and may require leave from duty. When it is mild, people often ignore it saying 'it's just a headache'. Thus, many times it goes undetected & untreated. In fact, most people don't consult a doctor for their headache and try to get relief by traditional or domestic methods but it is also an established fact that headache is the most common complaint for which people visit experts. Studies point out that headache is the 7th most common complaint for which patients see their family doctor. As a matter of fact, about 4% of all visits to doctors' office are because of headache.

The impact of headache cannot be minimized. Research has proved that amongst the reasons for which people miss their work, it stands out as the 3rd most common cause. Not only this, it makes very negative affect on the patients' personal and familial relationship. Patients suffering from serious Headache are unable to enjoy life.Their life becomes miserable. Thus, the quality of life of headache sufferers is very poor as compared with patients suffering from other chronic disorders.

Despite this, many people suffering from headache or migraine either ignore their headache or treat it themselves. Only about 50% of severe headache sufferers consult a doctor. This is because they think that either this is too mild problem or there is no remedy available.

Many famous personalities have been known to have suffered from serious Headache or Migraine. They include father of Psychiatry Sigmund Freud, Charles Darwin, Julius Caesar, Napoleon, Thomas Jefferson, Vincent Van Gogh, Pablo Picasso, Lewis Carroll and many others.

Headache is mostly of primary nature i.e., there is no physical reason behind it e.g. tension type headache, migraine and cluster headache but at times physical illness do cause headache which is then called secondary headache. Refractory error, cervical spondylitis, head injury, brain tumors, C.N.S. infections are a few examples. Therefore, in case of secondary headache, it becomes important to get proper investigations to be carried out for making correct diagnosis whereas for primary headache, investigations are of little help. A good history is sufficient to make right diagnosis. It has been seen that many patients of primary headache unnecessarily pressurize their doctors to get CT scan/ MRI and other investigations done. These are costly investigations and in the present scenario it is not available in small cities so these patients have to go to distant places for these investigations and in this process, a lot of money and time is lost. It is the doctor who is the best judge to decide when and what investigations are really required. So the patients of headache should have faith in their treating physicians, and should act as per their advice. Proper communication between the doctor and the patient is very important in the management of headache. The patients are required to give a coherent detail of their problem so that the doctor can have a clear view about the patient's symptoms of headache, about its frequency, duration and intensity, factors and circumstances which contribute or exaggerate their headache, under which conditions the headache gets reduced, previous treatment taken and the response with the medicines.

Among the primary type, tension type headache is the most common and we all are very familiar with this, as at least 80% of us face tension type headache at some point in our life. However, the most severe form of headache is migraine. It is a public health problem of enormous importance. It occurs in about 12% of the population. It can occur at any age. In children it is more common in boys, but after puberty it is much more common in girls. Even very young children suffer from it though making a diagnosis at this age is quite difficult unless they learn to speak. In women it is most common between the ages of 40 to 45. Men tend to develop migraine at a slightly younger age. Thus, it affects people in their most economically productive years.

Of the people with severe migraine 25% have 4 or more attacks in a month, 35% have 1- 4 attacks per month and 40% have <01 attack per month. Severe migraine leads to headache related disability in about 80-85% cases. About one-third of them could be severely disabled and need bed rest. These severe migraine sufferers live in perpetual fear of an attack even when there is no headache leading to disturbances in their career and relations. The disability thus caused is occasionally complete and it becomes impossible for the patients to carry on their work.

Migraine patients tend to use twice the medical resources including medicine and diagnostic tests every year as compared to non-migraineurs. The patients are so heavily distressed that they think that they are suffering from some serious medical disorder and it would be impossible for the doctor to pinpoint a correct diagnosis without detail proper investigations and hence they make repeated requests for these tests forcing doctors to order the investigations despite the fact that most of the time the doctor is sure that the investigations are of not much help.

Headache is rarely the first indication of a dangerous medical condition but a headache of sudden onset is worrisome. A better understanding of headaches will enable doctors to know when the patient of headache is serious enough to get properly investigated and treated accordingly and also to avoid unnecessary expensive investigations if he is sure of his diagnosis that the patient is suffering from primary headache.

❑❑

2
CHAPTER

History of Headache

Headache has been linked to the stress and speed of modern life but it is by no means a modern phenomenon. People have suffered from headaches since dawn of civilization and have been treating it. Some famous personalities who suffered from migraine are Sigmund Freud, Charles Darwin, Julius Caesar, Napoleon, Thomas Jefferson, Vincent Van Gogh, Pablo Picasso, Lewis Carroll and many others.

Attempts to treat serious headache dates back to as early as 7000 B.C. it was done by a procedure known as TREPANATION (perforating skull with an instrument). This practice is still followed by some African tribes and even in western societies. Reference to headache is found as far back as 3000 BC. In which headache triggers, relieving factors, signs and symptoms of migraine including headache, aura, nausea and/or vomiting have been described. The earliest public reference is a Sumerian epic poem which gives an early description of sickness by headache.

The Egyptians used Ebers Papyrus for headache treatment dating back 1200 BC. They believe like other ancients that the gods could cure their ailment if they followed divine instructions. They used to firmly bind a clay crocodile holding grain in its mouth to the patient's head by a strip of linen inscribed with the names of the gods. It may be assumed that the headache used to be relieved by compressing and cooling of the scalp.

Hippocrates 400 B.C. has described visual aura preceding migraine headache. He believed that headache could be triggered by exercise and sexual intercourse. He thought that migraine was a result of vapors rising from stomach to the head and vomiting could partially relieve the pain of headache.

The great philosopher Plato was of the view that preoccupation with the body triggered headaches. He said that excessive care of the body and always thinking about oneself results in dizziness and headache........' It makes the man always fancy himself sick and never cease from anguishing his body.' Thus, he emphasized the importance of one's aptitude and thinking in having or not having headache.

In ancient times, headache was considered to be a divine decree as a punishment for sins and curable by repentance and good deeds.

Celsius 215 -300 A.D. attributed 'drinking wine, or crudity (upset stomach), or cold, or heat of a fire or the Sun' could trigger migraine headache.

Migraine headache has been first described in 200 A.D. and the credit for this goes to Aretaeus of Cappodocia.

Galen 200 A.D. introduced the term 'Migraine' which is derived from Greek word 'Hemicrania', 'meaning by half of the head'. He mistakenly believed that it was caused by the ascent of vapors that were excessive, too hot or too cold. Later on, Migraine was also called by the names like Sick headache, Blind headache, Bilious headache.

The Europeans treated headache with application of a solution of Opium and Vinegar on skin in 13th century. Vinegar compresses have also been used alone as a headache treatment.

In late 1700s, Erasmus Darwin, grandfather of Charles Darwin, suggested vasodilatation as a cause of headache which is being still believed to be one of the important causative factors by some of the modern neurologists. He believed that placing the patient in a centrifuge would force the blood from head to feet thereby relieving headache.

Fothergill in 1778 introduced the term, 'fortification spectra' to describe visual aura or disturbance of migraine.

The first book on Migraine was written by Liveing in 1873, 'Megrine, sick headache, and some Allied Disorders: A contribution to the pathology of Nerve storms'. By nerve storms he meant problems originating due to disturbances of autonomic nervous system. He postulated the neural theory of migraine.

In 1888, William Gowers wrote, 'A Manual of disease of the nervous system'. He advocated the importance of a healthy lifestyle. This concept is now globally accepted not only for headache but also for cardiovascular diseases, diabetes, hypertension, backache, arthritis and psychiatric diseases etc. Gowers introduced a mixture of nitroglycerine 01% in alcohol along with other agents for the treatment of headache. This solution later became popular with the name of Gower's mixture. He also recommended Indian hemp (MARIJUANA) for headache relief.

Noted novelists like William Shakespeare in 'Othello', Stephen King in 'Fire Starter', Lewis Carroll in 'Alice in Wonderland' and 'Through the Looking Glass' have described symptoms of headache/Migraine to some extent.

Joan Didion in 'In Bed' has linked perfectionism with migraine personality.

General U.S. Grant in his Personal Memoirs has given a very clear-cut description that how emotional wellbeing can make dramatic change in headache intensity. On August 09, 1865 he suffered with intense sick headache which relieved only after Robert E. Lee surrendered. 'The instant I saw the contents of the note I was cured.'

The treatment of migraine became easier with the introduction of Ergotamine. Ergotamine is produced from Ergot, a fungus found on wheat and bread. Though it was already in use in obstetrics and gynecology, it was Rothlin who in 1925 for the first time successfully treated a case of severe and intractable migraine with a subcutaneous injection of Ergotamine tartrate.

John Graham and Harold Wolff in 1938, also used Ergotamine for treating headache and demonstrated that it worked by constricting blood vessels thus proving the vascular theory of migraine. Ergotamine proved to be a milestone in management of migraine. Later in1943 Dihydroergotamine (DHE) was synthesized by Stall and Hoffman and was used to treat migraine by Horton, Peters and Blumenthal.

Pat Humphrey and colleagues treated migraine with Sumatriptan based on the assumption that serotonin can relieve headache, they designed a chemical more stable than Serotonin but with fewer side effects. This development led to modern treatment of migraine. By now, 07 triptans have been developed and are being used for the treatment of headache

Thus, there has been tremendous change in the understanding, diagnosis and treatment of migraine and other headaches in recent years.

❑❑

3

CHAPTER

Causes and Triggers of Headache

It is important to know what causes headache for proper treatment. There is a difference between a cause and a trigger. A cause is directly responsible for headache while a trigger is only initiator of headache e.g., brain tumors, high fever, head injury can cause headache whereas stress and weather change act as trigger for primary headache.

Causes

TABLE - 1

- ❖ Brain Tumors
- ❖ High grade fever
- ❖ Head injury
- ❖ Infection like Meningitis and encephalitis
- ❖ Giant cell Arteritis

- Neck Disorders like Cervical spondylosis, Cervical Spondylitis
- Eye Problems like Refractory error
- ENT problems like Rhinosinusitis
- Trigeminal Neuralgia
- Dental problem like Temporomandibular disorder
- Severe Hypertension

Triggers

There are many factors which act as triggers of headache. Almost any physical problem in head and neck, including jaw joint, eyes, teeth and neck may be a trigger. Sometimes worsening of headache particularly migraine and to some extent tension type headache can be triggered by physical illness like viral fever, thyroid problem, sleep disturbances, chronic environmental factors like foul smell, psychological conditions like chronic stress and depression. Triggers play a little role in making cluster headache worse.

Triggers bring on the headaches one at a time and are not responsible for overall worsening of headache.

Here is a list of some common Migraine triggers:

TABLE - 2

Diet	Environmental Factors
Alcohol – Red Wine	Light glare
Caffeine withdrawal	Loud sound
Hunger	Odors
Additives	High altitude
Processed meat and fish	Weather change
Chinese Restaurant food	**Head or neck pain** (due to another cause)
Certain foods like ice-creams, cheese and other dairy products, chocolates	**Physical exertion:** Exercise Sex
	Stress and anxiety
Nuts, Onions, Beans, Pea Pods, Vinegar, Citrus Foods like Oranges, Lemon, Pineapple, Grapefruit	**Head trauma**
Sweeteners: - Asparmate	
Sleep Disturbances:	
Insomnia (decrease sleep)	
Hypersomnia (excessive sleep)	
Improper/Irregular Sleep schedule	

Hormonal Changes:	
Menstruation	
Thyroid disease	

Most red colored food trigger headache.

Food items containing Mono sodium glutamate, Nitrites and Nitrates, Tyramine do trigger headache.

Note: It is pointed out that individual items do not trigger headache in every individual. One item may be trigger to a patient but not to other patients.

❑❑

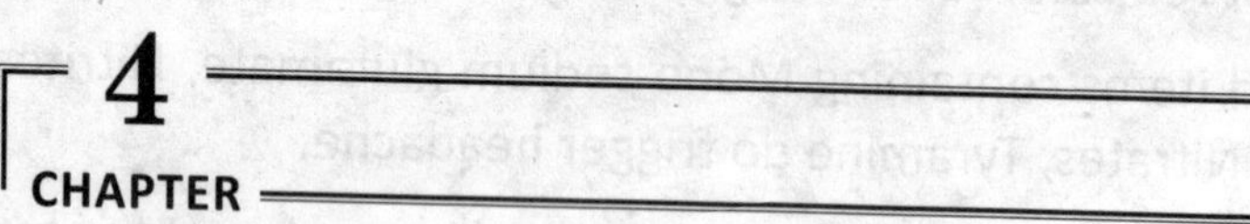

Certain Facts about Headache

Headache can be divided into two broad groups.

1. **Primary headache:** in this, the headache is itself a problem. There is no deeper underlying cause.
   a. Tension type headache – it is most common.
   b. Migraine – it is second most common.
   c. Cluster headache.
   d. Other rarer types include stabbing headache, cough headache, exertion headache, headache associated with sexual activity, hemi crania continua, new daily persistent headache etc.
2. **Secondary headache:** In this, the headache is a symptom of underlying conditions like brain tumor, stroke or fasting. To make a diagnosis, a

detailed history and proper physical examination is necessary. At times, if warning signs or any suspicious feature is present diagnostic tests may be required.

Most patients of headache have normal physical examination therefore the physician has to carry out detailed history of the patient like when and under what circumstances the headache appeared first and what has been its course? Migraine and tension type of headache usually begin in childhood or early adult life. Any new headache in middle age for the first time, say after 45 -50 years, is worrisome and may be a symptom of a serious disease. Headache with fever is suggestive of an infection.

A person can have more than one type of headache, and the pattern may change over time. The most important headache is the one that causes the most pain or the greatest worry to the sufferer.

While most headaches are not symptoms of a serious illness, some are.

Location and Duration of Pain

The pain of headache may be unilateral (one-sided) or bilateral (both sided). Migraine or Cluster headache and some unusual headaches are unilateral. Migraine pain can involve either side of head and may change sides in different attacks. It can even be bilateral, whereas pain of cluster headache is almost always one sided, with pain centered in or around the eye, temple, cheek or adjacent area, Tension type headache typically involves both sides of head.

In trigeminal neuralgia, there are jabs of brief, one-sided, severe pain (like electric current) on or near the upper or lower jaw or cheek that is triggered by light touch to a trigger zone lasting for few seconds and occurring many times a day. Headache due to neck diseases occur on the same side of disorder radiating from the neck to back of head.

In general, location of pain in primary headache is not very revealing. Establishing the headache profile is a critical factor in accurately diagnosing and properly treating headache.

Frequency and Timing of Attacks

Attacks of migraine occur at different times—for example on weekends, on vacations, related to menstruation, when relaxing after stress or at random. Cluster headache usually follow a regular pattern, occurring at similar times of day or night, often awakening the patient from sleep, one to three times a day during a cluster period, which usually lasts between two weeks and six month.

Duration of Headache

TABLE - 3

Type of Headache	Duration of attack
1. Trigeminal neuralgia	Seconds
2. Cluster headache	15 to 120 minutes
3. Migraine	4 to 72 hours
4. Status Migrainosus	>72 hours
5. Episodic Tension type	30 minutes to 7 days

For enabling the doctor to make a correct diagnosis the patient must give detailed account of the frequency and timing of headache including mild as well as severe attacks of headache or daily headache.

Pain Severity and Quality

The severity and the speed of onset and resolution of pain are important diagnostic clues. Headache of sudden onset is worrisome. Severity of pain is measured by asking the patient to mark it on a 1 to 10 scale with 1 representing minimum discomfort and 10 as the most excruciating pain the person has suffered. The patient must be honest in such measurements. Over exaggeration like marking as 15/10 serves no purpose. Rather it confuses the doctor and the patient loses credibility. Consistency is very important, so that both the doctor and the patient can know about the progress being made in the treatment.

Tension type headache is usually dull aching, turban band like. There is a feeling of heaviness in head.

Migraine pain is typically throbbing or pulsating type, but it can begin as dull, steady, and slowly progress to severe throbbing type.

Cluster headache pain is deep, boring, or piercing described as though a red-hot poker were being thrust into the eye.

Associated Features

Migraine attacks are usually associated with nausea and/ or vomiting. Even diarrhea may occur. Such patients are highly sensitive to light and sound.

Cluster headache is associated with eye-tearing, redness, congestion of nose and occasionally swelling of face on the side of headache.

Factors Influencing Headache

There are certain factors which initiate or worsen headache. They are actual triggers. For example ,if someone develops muscle pull in shoulder or neck, he gets an attack of migraine. Here the neck pain due to muscle pull acts as a migraine trigger. There may be other triggers as well but when neck problem is serious, the migraine is more severe. Removing the trigger is important but one must not get confused and say that the problem is strictly in the neck. Menstruation is a common trigger for many women. Alcohol is also a well-known trigger.

In case of Trigeminal Neuralgia there are several trigger points on the face and the mouth. If these trigger points are stimulated even slightly by touching, stroking, shaving, washing the face or eating, brushing the teeth, even speaking or exposure to cold may induce an attack.

Sleep disturbances like sleep apnea (a condition where breathing is stopped for some time during sleep, then patient partially awakens), sleep deprivation (as happens when one attends marriage ceremonies or in late night parties or seeing television or cinema till late night) also act as triggers of migraine headache particularly in morning.

Life style stressors (like marriage, employment status, education, retirement, birth or death in a family, children going abroad or distant places, separation, disputes, court cases, poor working conditions, over burden with work, job dissatisfaction, inter-personal problems etc.) play important role in producing chronic headache.

A good night's sleep often clears the attack. Migraine patients seek relief by retiring to a dark, quiet room lying motionless on bed. Hot and cold compressions and pressure on the head relieves the headache temporarily. The frequency and severity of migraine pain is significantly reduced during the last two trimesters of pregnancy and following menopause.

Relaxation, rest, engaging oneself in some activity or distraction often helps the patients of Tension-type headache.

Cluster headache patients often sit upright, rock in a chair, pace to and fro, and engage in vigorous movement in order to get some relief.

Family History

Headache is often seen running in families. Not only this, the pattern of headache is also similar in many instances. Nearly 50-60% migraine patients have a parent with the disorder and about 80% have at least one first degree relative with migraine. Approximately 50% patients of Tension Type headache have family members with similar headache. Cluster headaches rarely occur within the same family.

It is not only the genetic factor responsible for familial headache but some environmental exposure may also bring on similar headache. For example, a malfunctioning furnace may cause carbon monoxide –induced headaches in an entire family.

How Headache Affects a Person's Life?

The impact of headache differs in different individuals. For some it is decapitating. Headache affects personal, social, family, and leisure activity. His work performance in office, home, or school deteriorates. To measure the level of activity limitation, doctors may use migraine disability assessment (MIDAS) questionnaire. It can measure actual days of missed activity – for example, work absenteeism and the number of days with high levels of activity limitation. It can help both doctors and patients focus on how headache affects a person's life. A MIDAS score greater than 10 indicates significant disability. Headache impact test (HIT) – 6 is another test which assesses emotional impact as well as physical disability.

Migraine is the likely diagnosis when there is a high level of disability due to a recurrent (comes and goes) primary headache.

Physical and Neurological Examination

It is important for the physician to take a thorough history of the patient and do proper physical (including neurological) examination. He should check pulse, blood pressure, base line weight. He should also examine heart and lungs and blood vessels in the neck. The head and neck examination is important to look for any growth, bruises, tenderness, trigger points and thickened blood vessels. Jaw movements should also be checked.

The doctor must see the fundus of the eyes to check for any signs of Papilledema which may suggest a possibility of a space occupying lesion in the brain like a brain tumor. Any weakness in arms or legs or facial paralysis suggests a disease in the brain. A thickened or nodular scalp artery, diminished or absent artery pulsations, red tender scalp nodules, or necrotic lesions of the scalp or tongue suggest giant cell arteritis (also known as temporal arteritis), a cause of headache and sudden blindness in elderly people.

Many a time, it is difficult to make a clear-cut diagnosis on the first visit. The initial diagnosis may even be incorrect. Therefore, it is being suggested that both the doctors and the patients should re-evaluate the first diagnosis and for this the patient should be asked to maintain a headache diary mentioning about the timings, intensity, severity and nature of headache including any possible trigger as well as response to the treatment given so that the unrecognized patterns of headache may be uncovered and give clue to diagnosis.

Investigations

Most of the patients with headache don't need any test to confirm the diagnosis as they suffer from primary type headache like tension headache or migraine. There are certain factors which indicate that that the headaches are not due to an underlying organic cause. They are:

Reassuring Factors

TABLE - 4

❖ Headache occurring at a regular or near regular hormonal timing e.g., menstruation
❖ Headache occurring after sustained exertion
❖ Relief with sleep
❖ Food, odor, or weather changes provoking headache

In case of school going children and young adults, headache may be caused by eye problems like decreased vision (refractory error) for which a simple test of refraction is to be carried out. Middle aged people occasionally have neck problem like cervical spondylitis for which x-ray of neck is to be done.

Diagnostic tests are required if the doctor suspects or wants to rule out a serious underlying condition like stroke, brain tumor or subdural hematoma etc. Some baseline tests are helpful prior to treatment. They are—blood investigations like complete blood count (CBC) & liver function test (LFT), electrocardiogram (ECG) may be done before starting medication. Erythrocyte sedimentation rate (ESR) measures inflammation in the body and can establish the diagnosis of giant cell arteritis.

Computed tomography (CT) and Magnetic Resonance imaging (MRI) are useful for atypical headaches which do not fit into any defined primary headache- for example, they are used to rule out the possibility of a brain tumor. However, CT and MRI are not required in patients of migraine if there has been no change in the pattern of headache in the recent past, no history of seizure, no signs of a focal neurological deficit like weakness in any limb.

Though electroencephalogram (EEG) is usually of not much help but sometimes it becomes difficult to differentiate between symptoms of migraine aura and symptoms of epilepsy which are similar then EEG may be of some help to make a correct diagnosis.

As CT or MRI may miss presence of blood or infection, Lumbar Puncture is needed. So even, when CT or MRI is normal, Lumbar Puncture may be required. Lumbar puncture (LP) also known as spinal tap (a procedure in which a needle is placed in between two vertebrae and a fluid known as cerebrospinal fluid is taken out and is sent for analysis) is done to measure the pressure of fluid and to determine whether an infection is present or not. It is done in following indications—

Indications for Lumbar Puncture

TABLE - 5

- The first or worst headache of life
- Severe, rapid onset, recurrent headache
- Progressive headache (over days or weeks)
- A typical, chronic intractable headache
- Daily headache with symptoms of high spinal fluid pressure
- Headache with fever (meningitis)

❑❑

5

CHAPTER

When is Headache Serious Enough to Seek Medical Help?

In the OPD, patients of headache often describe their problem like 'Doctor, please save me. It seems that my head is going to explode. Please, get my CT done. It looks as if I have got a brain tumor.'

Often such patients who have their first severe headache are frightened and think of dire consequences, but fortunately such incidences are rare. Headache is rarely the first indication of a dangerous medical condition. But, if it is, when should one definitely seek immediate medical help? The below table illustrates certain warning signs which may act as a guide-line for identifying serious conditions.

TABLE - 6

Some Important Cacts:

- Most of the headaches are not a symptom of a serious disease (except a few)
- Most of the time, physical examination of the patient's of headache is within normal limit. hence history of headache, when and under what cicumstances it happens is more important.
- The most important headache is that which is most serious or for which the patient is most concerned.
- Headache appearing for the first time in a patient of over 45-50 years of age or a new headache or a change in pattern of headache may be a symptom of a serious illness like a brain tumor. such patients should be investigated with ct or mri.
- Headache associated with fever is due to infection.

Alarming Signs

TABLE - 7

- Sudden onset or 'thunderclap' headache.
- A marked change in headache pattern, it's frequency, severity and duration.

- ❖ Neurologic signs and symptoms like double vision, blindness, confusion, dizziness, weakness, loss of sensations.
- ❖ Signs of meningitis like painful and stiff neck.
- ❖ Symptoms of brain damage like weakness of one side of body (paralysis).
- ❖ Unexplained fever.
- ❖ Persistent or recurrent vomiting.
- ❖ Head injury.
- ❖ Convulsions.
- ❖ Progressive Worsening of headache.
- ❖ B.P. >180/115 mm hg.
- ❖ Headache appearing for the first time after 45-50 years of age.

Serious Medical Conditions Causing Severe Headache

Sub Arachnoid Hemorrhage

This is a very serious condition. In this, bleeding occurs under the membrane that surrounds the brain due to rupture of aneurysm (bulge in a blood vessel due to weak walls of the blood vessel). The headache is sudden, very intense, reaching its peak in about one minute only. This is a real, life threatening emergency. Many patients die before reaching hospital. Even with best care, many die or suffer stroke. Immediate neurosurgical intervention can save lives and prevent complications like future stroke.

Giant Cell Arteritis (Temporal Arteritis)

(Arteritis means inflammation of blood vessels)

In this, the patient, usually an elderly (twice as common in females as in males), presents with headache with scalp tenderness over an artery along with general feeling of being sick, pain in muscles and joints, low grade fever, depression and some visual disturbance. Stroke may also happen. There may be necrotic lesions of scalp or tongue. The combination of new – onset headache, jaw claudication, and abnormal (nodular or tender) arteries is highly predictive. On examination, there may be diminished or absent temporal artery pulsations.

ESR is invariably raised (more than 30 mm/hr.).

Meningitis and Encephalitis

Meningitis means inflammation of surface (meninges) of brain while Encephalitis means inflammation of the substances of brain, not just the coverings. It is caused by infection mostly viral or bacterial. There is an alarming increase in cases of encephalitis in the recent past in eastern U.P. particularly Gorakhpur division. With media focus, it has not only scared general public but also the politicians leading to agitations, forcing both the central and state governments to establish a virology and encephalitis Centre in the state at Gorakhpur.

The patient is very serious, presenting with symptoms of headache, nausea and vomiting along with fever, sensitivity to light and sound. The neck of the patient becomes stiff, he starts losing consciousness, as the condition deteriorates. He develops attacks of seizures (convulsions) i.e., abnormal bodily movements, along with psychiatric symptoms like abnormal behavior. There may be problems of speech and language. Studies have revealed that about one-fifth to one-sixth of the patients die despite treatment. Among those who survive develop handicap (both physical as well as mental). Most of them usually become mentally retarded. Very few patients are lucky enough to have no residual symptoms.

The patients need proper investigations like Lumbar Puncture, CT or MRI Scan apart from other routine investigations.

Brain Tumor

The word 'brain tumor' shakes people too much. The general public is so frightened that even if the patient is suffering from primary type of headache like migraine or tension type headache, they want to know whether their headache is a symptom of a brain tumor or not. That's why there is a great demand from patient and their family's side for investigations like CT or MRI to be done despite it being a very expensive investigation.

The headaches caused by brain tumor usually resemble headache of migraine or tension type headache but may be of different variety as well. It may even be worse than the headache of primary type. Though the headache of a brain tumor may awaken him from sleep but such morning headaches are not usually due to brain tumors. There are other reasons also for morning headaches. It is also important to understand that patients of brain tumors also have several other symptoms along with headache. For example, it is often associated with weakness, loss of vision, fever, decreased appetite, clumsiness of the limbs, difficulty in walking, abnormal sensation in one side of body. Even seizures may present. The headache as the only symptom is rare in case of a brain tumor.

It is interesting to note that about more than half the patients suffering from brain tumors have headache and about 80% of those have pain on the same side of tumor. Sometimes, patients of brain tumors have mild pain in the beginning but it may worsen over a period of few days or weeks. As the brain tumor usually occurs in later years of life, the doctor should be cautious when seeing patients of more than 50 years of age.

There is a condition that looks like a tumor but it is not, is known as pseudo tumor. In this, there is increased spinal fluid pressure; usually there are signs of swelling in the back of the eye and temporary visual symptoms also. This headache is relieved by a spinal tap. The patient feels so comfortable with this that he even asks for another one!

Hypertension

Headaches are usually not caused by high blood pressure unless it is very high i.e., when the diastolic blood pressure (lower side) is more than 115 mm hg. Such a high B.P. is a medical emergency.

Some people with migraine headache respond to drugs used in high B.P. so, when such a person's blood pressure medicine is stopped, headache may occur, giving the impression that high blood pressure causes headache.

Dissection (Rupture of the Lining of an Artery)

In this, the lining of an artery supplying blood to the brain gets ruptured and the blood enters the wall of the artery expanding it, there by obstructing the blood flow to the brain leading to intense headache which appears similar to migraine with aura. It may be accompanied by stroke-like symptoms like weakness, numbness, blindness, and inability to speak. This condition may persist for more than 24 hours.

Post Spinal tap Headache and other Low-pressure Headaches

In case of encephalitis and meningitis, a procedure known as spinal tap (lumbar puncture) is done to confirm the diagnosis. In this, a needle is placed in the spine in the lower back and the spinal fluid is taken out and is sent for analysis in pathology lab. Rarely does it lead to long term complications and permanent injury. But in about 10% cases, due to persistent leakage of spinal fluid through a hole in the coverings of spinal cord, headache develops. This is called post-spinal headache. The patient develops headache as soon as (within seconds or minutes) he stands up. The headache disappears as he lies down. The headache usually starts in back of head or upper part of the neck and spreads over the entire head. It is not associated with any kind of nausea or light/sound sensitivity. Although doctors advise the patients to lie down for hours following spinal tap (lumbar puncture), this doesn't protect him from getting the post spinal tap headache.

Usually, this headache improves of its own over several days. The patient is advised to lie flat and drink plenty of fluids. An abdominal binder may be helpful. Caffeine oral or intravenous is helpful if given rapidly. Blood patch, a procedure, may need to be done. In this procedure a patient's own blood is withdrawn and injected into a space surrounding the spinal cord. This procedure gives wonderful results instantly. It is said that this is successful in 98% cases.

❑❑

6

CHAPTER

Migraine

Migraine has been defined by "The Ad Hoc Committee on Classification of Headache" as "recurrent attacks of headache, widely varied in intensity, frequency and duration. The attacks are commonly unilateral in onset, are usually associated with loss of appetite and sometimes, with nausea and vomiting, in some they are preceded by or associated with conspicuous sensory, motor and move disturbances and they are often familial".

The migraine attacks are usually severe, last from 4 hours to 72 hours, is a pulsating or throbbing type, often unilateral but at times it is bilateral as well. Many times, these attacks subside after vomiting. At times it is preceded by Aura i.e., colored halos floating in front of eyes, tingling or numbness in limbs, abnormal smell or hearing of voices etc. Besides these, dizzy spells, tinnitus, weakness in limbs and fainting attacks etc. may occur.

It occurs in about 12% of population (18% females and 6% males) in any given year. It may happen at any age. In childhood, it is more common in boys but after puberty girls outnumber boys. It tends to start earlier in boys (around 10 years age) than the girls (around 15 years age). Though even small children may have migraine headache, but it is very difficult to make a diagnosis at this age. They usually present as recurrent vomiting or dizzy spells. The child may have activity-affected headache (he may be motionless/lie down/sleep off). The common migraine triggers in children are—sun exposure, travelling by bus, missing meals, strenuous physical exercise, and sleep disturbance. Usually one family member, particularly the mother is also suffering from migraine.

Recent studies have confirmed that children, who have adverse lipid profile, are likely to develop migraine in adulthood. Thus, adverse lipid profile in childhood is a risk factor for migraine in adulthood.

In ladies, it is more common at 40-45 years of age, while the males develop migraine at a relatively younger age. Thus, it affects people mostly in their economically productive years. After menopause its frequency decreases. In the elderly, severe nausea with migraine tends to decrease, and at times have only aura and no headache. This is called 'migraine equivalents of the elderly.' They are difficult to be differentiated from transient ischemic attacks (may be a warning spell for stroke).

About 25% patients having severe migraine have more than four attacks in one month while about 35% have one to four attacks per month and about 40% patients have less than one attack in a month. 80-85% people with severe migraine become disabled and about one-third of them have to take rest in bed. They are in constant fear that they will develop headache attack again. This puts a bad impact on their career as well as in their personal relations. They have to skip social meetings; thereby they are unable to enjoy the pleasures of life. Their life becomes dull and boring. A recent study reports that a migraine attack diminishes cognitive performance like a learning defect. It suggests that there is a reversible cortical dysfunction in the pre-frontal and temporal brain areas during the migraine without aura attacks.

Migraineurs use medical facilities twice than non-migraineurs. Till now no known cause has been identified for migraine to happen, however it is assumed that migraine occurs as a result of inflammations in vessels of brain leading to leakage of certain neuro-chemicals which make the brain sensitive and thereby producing pain. Migraine has also got some relation with hormones, as in case with females, it is more common during menstruation and it disappears after menopause.

The patients of migraine demand investigations, but there is no test for it. The tests, if conducted at all, are done only to rule out other causes of headache or to satisfy the patient psychologically, so that he may be convinced that he is not suffering from any dangerous condition. Otherwise, no tests are actually required. Here lies the importance of patient's faith in the doctor. The more faith the patient is, in his doctor, the more are the chances of the patient to believe the diagnosis of the doctor, thereby not insisting on their demand for unwarranted investigations, thus limiting the expenditure.

About 1.5-2.0% people with migraine become chronic i.e., they have migraine attacks more than 15 days in a month.

The attacks may be controlled with drugs like NSAIDS (Non-Steroid Anti Inflammatory Drugs) or opioids/steroids/antinauseants or with specific drugs like ergotamines, dihydroergotamine, and triptans like sumatriptans-which is more effective. For prophylaxis β blockers, anti-depressants, calcium channel blockers like verapamil, flunarazine, Neuro modulators like divalproex sodium, topiramate and others like butox etc. are used.

Classification of Migraine

In early 1980s, the International Headache Society (IHS) classified migraine into several types, the most important being migraine without aura and migraine with aura.

Migraine without Aura

Previously it was known as common migraine.

TABLE - 8

International classification of headache disorders – 3 Beta version [ICHD-3 beta] Diagnostic criteria for migraine without aura
A. At least five attacks fulfilling criteria B-D B. Headache attacks lasting 4-72 h (untreated or unsuccessfully treated) C. Headache has at least two of the following four characteristics: ❖ Unilateral Location ❖ Pulsating quality ❖ Moderate or severe pain intensity ❖ Aggravation by or causing avoidance of routine physical activity (e.g., walking or climbing stairs) D. During headache at least one of the following: ❖ Nausea and/or vomiting ❖ Photophobia and Phonophobia E. Not better accounted for by another ICHD-3 beta diagnosis

"Manju is a 29 year old working lady. She visited her psychiatrist for her headaches which used to disturb her frequently since she was a student of high school. She reported that she develops headache mostly one sided, but of late, occasionally she is having headache on both sides. She describes that she feels her head is going to explode. It lasts for several hours. Usually, she feels as if she will vomit out (nauseated). Sometimes she has vomiting and then there is rapid relief and she feels quite relaxed. She has also noticed that whenever she goes out in Sun without covering her head, she develops these attacks. The attacks also occur when she attends marriage parties where there is lot of noise due to music systems and bright flashing lights. Initially the headache occurred once in two months but its frequency has increased. Now she is having once every 10 days. On an average she has to miss her work once or twice a month. The regular headache subsided with analgesics like paracetamol, but the severe ones never subside soon. She has consulted several physicians but could not get much relief. She even got MRI done which was normal. Now she has been referred to the psychiatrist."

Manju is suffering from Migraine without Aura.

The IHS defines headache without aura as headache that last for few hours, on one side of head, pulsating quality, and moderate to severe intensity, interfering with normal daily activity and is associated with nausea/ vomiting and/or sensitivity to light or sound. Not all of the above symptoms are present but at least some of them are necessary for the diagnosis of Migraine without Aura.

TABLE - 9

To understand migraine without aura the salient features are as following: The headache, when treated or untreated, but without improvement—lasts from 4 to 72 hours, and at least two of the following characteristics are present:
1. The headache is only on one side. 2. The headache is of pulsating quality. 3. The pain is moderate or severe and interferes with normal daily activity. 4. The pain is aggravated by walking stairs or similar physical activity. During the headache, at least one of the following is present: 1. Nausea and /or vomiting. 2. Photophobia (light sensitivity) and phonophobia (sound sensitivity) The headache is not caused by any other disorder.

TABLE - 10

The most distinguished symptoms of migraine can be remembered by the mnemonics 'POUND', as in 'a pounding headache'.

- ❖ P – pulsatile quality (headache described as pounding or throbbing)
- ❖ O – one day duration (episode of headache lasts 4-72 hours if untreated)
- ❖ U – unilateral location
- ❖ N –nausea or vomiting
- ❖ D – disabling intensity (headache disables the patient to carry out usual daily activity)

The pain increases with movement. The pain is supposed to be one-sided, but in about 40% cases, it is present on both sides of head. Some patients may be sensitive to even odors.

Some Migraineurs complain about nasal congestion, but the fact is that most people with "sinus headache" actually suffer from migraine. They do not have any disorder of nasal passage or sinus. Similarly, many patients of migraine have complaints of pain in upper neck along with it or before or after the headache.

Migraine with Aura

Previously it was known as classic migraine.

TABLE - 11

International classification of headache disorders – 3 Beta version [ICHD-3 beta]
Diagnostic criteria for migraine with aura

Diagnostic Criteria:
A. At least two attacks fulfilling criteria B and C B. One or more of the following fully reversible aura Symptoms: ❖ Visual ❖ Sensory ❖ Speech and/or language ❖ Retinal C. At least two of the following four characteristics: ❖ At least one aura symptom spreads gradually over 5 minutes, and/or two or more ❖ Each individual aura symptom lasts 5-60 min ❖ At least one aura symptom is unilateral ❖ The aura is accompanied or followed within 60 min by headache. D. Not better accounted for by another ICHD-3 beta diagnosis, and transient ischemic attack has been excluded.

In Migraine with Aura, there is a physical warning before the headache develops. The warning is in form of something floating in front of eyes or some visual hallucination or some sensory or other central nervous system symptoms (speech/language, motor or brainstem or retinal). These symptoms are unilateral, develop gradually and are fully reversible usually followed by headache and other migraine symptoms. Normally they last for 20 minutes.

"Ravi, a 25-year-old research scholar, was driving his car. He suddenly noticed a spot in front of his eyes which was surrounded with twinkling light and was floating in air. He had to stop his car. The spot grew larger and then disappeared. This visual phenomenon occurred for about 10-15 minutes only followed by mild headache lasting for half an hour. In the last 6 months he had similar problem on at least three occasions. His brother also has similar problem. He consulted his doctor, who diagnosed him to be suffering from migraine with aura. Ravi asked for a CT scan but the doctor convinced him about the mild nature of illness and told that a scan was not warranted. He was reassured and sent home."

Obviously, Ravi is suffering from Migraine with aura.

Basilar Migraine is another type of migraine with aura. In this, the aura (symptoms preceding headache) is in the form of double vision, dizzy spells (vertigo), ringing in ears, unsteady gait, and altered consciousness, even fainting at times. This type of migraine with aura is more common in teen aged girls but may occur at any age.

"Neeta was an 18 year old college girl. She was participating in a group discussion. Suddenly she started staring and everything appeared to her as double. This lasted for about 1 minute. She felt dizzy; the room appeared to be spinning and then she fainted. After a few minutes she woke up. Now she was having severe headache. She described that her head was hurt all over. She had an episode of vomiting. She could not stand or walk properly for few minutes. Her headache persisted for hours. She had another attack after 10 days."

Neeta is suffering from basilar migraine.

Cause of Migraine

Many theories have been postulated from nerve storms of 1870s to vascular theory in 1950s, but none could give a complete understanding about migraine. In 1970s, the serotonin theory was developed. It was suggested that migraine occurred as a result of imbalance in serotonin function. Serotonin is a neurotransmitter which transmits impulses from one nerve to another. In the 1990s, neurogenic inflammation theory was considered. It stated that migraine was a result of inflammation of blood vessels and the lining of brain; the most current theory is neurovascular theory. It is being understood that migraine is a brain disorder that affects the blood vessels. During a migraine attack, chemicals are released from nerve endings which lead to leakage from blood vessels. The nerve endings are responsible for the head pain, but the other symptoms are derived from brain.

Despite all these theories, we are not able to pin point a single factor. Perhaps there are multiple factors responsible for migraine. At least five facts have been identified that may cause headache. They are:

1. It has been noticed that the brains of migraineurs are very sensitive and are hyper excitable. They behave differently than non migraineurs. Recently it has been discovered that the migraineurs see a flash of light at a significantly lower power pulse than do non-migraineurs. This indicates that the visual part of migraineurs brain is hypersensitive. Similarly, if an alternating checkerboard is shown over a period of time, the amplitude of their brain wave response tends to increase in migraineurs whereas the non-migraineurs tend to show a decrease in the amplitude of this wave as they get used to it. This suggests that the brain's response to recurrent stimuli is different in the migraineurs.
2. The aura of migraine is caused by a wave of increased electrical activity that moves across the surface of the brain, followed by a loss of activity. Initially there is increased blood flow for a brief period which is followed by a period of decreased blood flow. The increased brain activity causes the bright lights seen in typical visual aura and the decreased brain activity causes visual loss – either a gray, dark, or white area that the person cannot see through.

3. There are certain specific areas in the brain which are activated in migraine. They may be called the "migraine generators". They are supposed to be located in the upper brain stem. Inputs from emotional and sensory areas are received here and from here impulses are sent back to these areas. Fibers carrying pain information reach the center of the brain in this area, and the area of brain considered to be the migraine generator have connections with the pain center that receive information from the blood vessels.

4. The throbbing pain of migraine is thought to be due to inflammation of the covering of the brain (meninges) or blood vessels. Such Inflammation occurs because of a mechanical or electrical stimulation. Nerve endings secrete inflammatory proteins around meninges and vessels. The blood vessels dilate and leak, and the nerve endings on blood vessels and meninges become more reactive causing throbbing pain.

   Magnetic Resonance Angiography (MRA) study has revealed that there is slight dilatation of intracranial arteries (internal carotid artery) during a migraine attack.

5. The migraineurs are so sensitive that at times even non painful stimulation of scalp or other

parts of head or even arms result in development of a migraine attack. This is known as allodynia. The patient also feels increased pain on bending, straining, or shaking the head. There is tenderness (pain on touch) of scalp and neck, combing hair is painful. Patient tends to avoid cold or hot wind in hair. She finds jewelries to be causing pain, so takes them off and loosen their collar. Allodynia usually develops after 4 to 6 hours of start of migraine attack. It is very difficult to treat migraine once allodynia is established.

Symptoms of migraine

'Complete Migraine' is the most appropriate term to understand all the symptoms of migraine. There are four stages: the prodrome, the aura, the headache, and the postdrome.

The prodrome or the premonitory symptoms occur from hours to one day before the actual headache. The patient presents with many descriptions non-painful behaviors and feelings. He feels depressed and slows down in all activity. There may be food cravings and increased appetite. Many patients who like chocolate, start taking it too much. That's why chocolate has been falsely identified as a trigger of migraine. There may be mood swings, often irritability. The patient may also have much yawning.

The aura is present in about 20% of migraineurs. It may not be present in all headaches. It is of many types. Mostly it is the visual aura in the form of scintillating scotoma (a bright area of flashing lights appear over center or to the right or left side of one's area of central vision, expanding over in about 20 minutes in one side of visual field). The lights are white or yellow or any other color flashing bright. As it migrates across the visual field, it leaves a scotoma, an area of decreased vision in form of black, gray, white, or clear area. The visual aura is usually bilateral but may be unilateral as well.

The second most common type of aura is sensory aura, during which tingling or numbness occurs in one hand or lips spreading in the upper limbs.

There are certain other auras like inability to speak normally (Aphasia), weakness of one side of body, or hallucinations of abnormal smells. Rarely in children there is visual distortions and alterations in perspective of body image. It is called the "Alice in Wonderland syndrome."

Auras may occur one after another. The patient may have a typical visual aura, followed by a sensory aura, then an aphasic aura and finally a motor aura. Some patients have a time gap between the end of an aura and beginning of headache. The thinking process in this period may not be normal.

Headache is the 3rd stage. Usually, it is like migraine without aura: throbbing, pulsating, or severe pain on one side of head getting worse on movement, associated with nausea, vomiting and increased sensitivity to light and sound. The pain may spread to both sides. There may be other symptoms like pale, clammy skin, slight swelling of fingers, feet and face. They may have thinking and behavioral problems like difficulty in concentration and memory, slight decline in alertness. They find difficulty in writing correctly. Most patients want to be left alone. Many patients suffer from Allodynia (sensitive to otherwise pleasant or non-painful touch). They complain that their head hurts on brushing hair. They are unable to lay their painful side of head on pillow, take off jewelry, loosen their collars, avoid air blowing on the head, avoid cold or heat applied onto the scalp.

Some patients get relief from pain in a peculiar way: there may be an elimination of a large amount of urine, bowel movement or vomiting with an abrupt sense of release in the head and the pain is gone in few minutes. A few patients even induce vomiting to relieve severe headache.

Postdrome is the final stage. The patient has feelings or sensations which are out of proportion to the severity of pain. They often complain of tiredness and depression. There may be unusual joy that is more than expected from the simple relief that the headache is gone.

Migraine and Menstrual & Hormonal Changes

Some relationship between migraine and sex hormones estrogen and progesterone has been observed. Migraine begins or increases dramatically at the onset of puberty and generally improves after menopause. Many women tend to have their most severe migraine around the time of menses. The most distinctive form of menstrual migraine occurs just after the onset of flow and appears to be due to the sudden drop in the estrogen levels that occurs around the menses. The brain's abnormal response to normal hormonal fluctuations determines whether a woman will develop menstrual migraine. Such women benefit with replacement with estrogen. Some women have premenstrual migraine headache associated with premenstrual syndrome. Many women with regular migraine report worsening of their headache around or during their periods. Menstrual migraine is difficult to treat, but this is not with all cases. NSAIDs and frovatriptan are effective for short term prevention of menstrual migraine.

Oral contraceptives are relatively safe for women younger than 35 years age who have migraine without aura. Women with intractable menstrual migraine are good candidates for a trial of oral contraceptives. World Health Organization (WHO) discourage use of estrogen containing contraceptives in women having Migraine with aura and urge caution for those having migraine without aura and are older than 35 years or have other risk factors like smoking, obesity, or hypertension.

In some cases, migraine tends to worsen during menopause. Estrogen replacement is beneficial, but it should be used judiciously after a natural menopause.

Migraine and Pregnancy

Migraine improves during pregnancy in about 60 to 70 % of women, mostly in the second and third semester. As most drugs have not been proved to be safe in pregnancy, they should be better avoided. Rather, non-pharmacologic treatment should be the mainstay of migraine management. In a study , about 80% of pregnant women showed significant relief when treated with physical therapy, relaxation training, and biofeedback. The beneficial effect was maintained for up to a year after delivery.

The pregnant women and their family members should be reassured that migraine is a benign condition and that there is no significant impact on the mother or fetus during pregnancy.

Migraine and Breast-Feeding

Following child birth, just over half of the women with migraine, have recurrence of headache in the first month after delivery. However, in women who breast feed their child, chances of the recurrence are delayed. Most studies support that breast feeding acts as a protective measure against migraine. Acetaminophen and ibuprofen are the safest analgesics for breast feeding women. It has been categorized as compatible by American academy of pediatrics and Briggs category. Other drugs which have been identified as compatible and can be used by breast feeding mothers for migraine are-indomethacin, ketorolac, naproxen, eletriptan, caffeine, prednisone and prednisolone. Some other drugs which have been categorized as probably compatible include Gabapentin (antiepileptic), antihypertensives like Timolol, Candesartan, Labetalol, Lisnopril and Verapamil. Hormonal contraceptives, estrogen – estradiol, melatonin, riboflavin, magnesium sulphate and cyproheptadine are also probably compatible.

Migraine and Stroke

Migraine and stroke are the most common disorders affecting adults. Migraine, particularly with aura, is associated with increased stroke risk both during and between attacks. As such, migraine may be viewed as a potentially modifiable risk factor for stroke. The exact mechanism by which migraine can predispose to stroke is not certain. Acute stroke and migraine aura usually share a common pathophysiology of cortical spreading depression (CSD). Individuals suffering from migraine are predisposed to CSD, they are also at a risk of developing larger acute infarcts.

Migraine and Obesity

There is an association between migraine and obesity. Though obesity does not cause migraine, it promotes its frequency. Normal weight people with migraine have about a 3% chance of developing chronic migraine in a year. Overweight people have 3 times and obese people have 5 times chance of developing chronic migraine as compared to normal weight persons with migraine.

In both obesity and migraine, multiple pain generating hormones are released including calcitonin gene related peptide, substance p, tumor necrosis factor α, and interleukin-6. Thus, the release of these chemicals from the 2 sources predisposes obese persons with migraine to have more headaches. Similarly, both obese and migraine patients have higher levels of insulin, glucose and plaque promoting LDL cholesterol than in the general population, thus increasing the risk of heart attack and stroke in obese patients with migraine.

Therefore, reducing weight is important for successful management of chronic migraine.

Migraine and Vitamin D

There is a report that links migraine to a vitamin D deficiency. Though it is not clear whether the vitamin D deficiency is a cause or a consequence of migraine. Chronic migraine patients have been found to have lower levels of vitamin D versus episodic migraine patients.

Migraine and its Timing

People develop migraine at different times. While some are awakened by it early in the morning (most common time for migraine to develop), others have migraine in middle of day which gets worsened in the evening (during working hours). There are still some persons who do not have migraine during a very active work week when they are much stressed, but they are awakened in the early morning of the weekend with severe migraine headache along with nausea and vomiting, thereby debilitating him and ruining his holiday. This paradox can be explained by –

1. Due to the ongoing stress during the working days headache was building up which was expressed because of let-down or release of stress.
2. Over sleeping in weekends/holidays, as oversleeping acts as a trigger for headache.

3. Caffeine/tea withdrawal since first cup of coffee or tea may be taken late in weekends/holidays.

Maintaining the weekend schedule similar to other days, getting up and taking coffee/tea at routine time, may help.

Some patients have seasonal headaches – either in winters or in summers only. Thus, for no reasonable explanation, this seasonal trend in such patients has been established.

❑❑

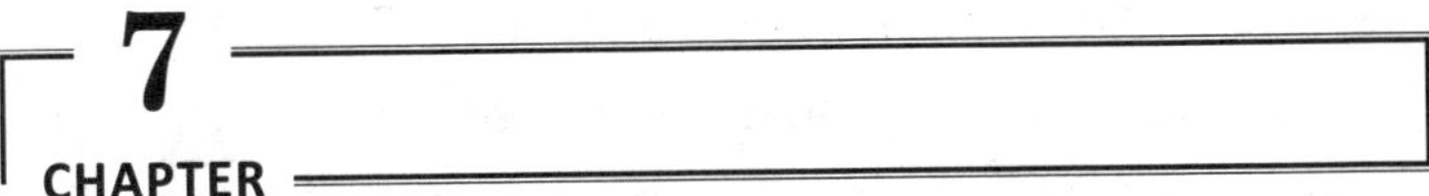

7 CHAPTER

Chronic Headache

When headaches of migraine occur more than 15 days in a month it is called 'chronic headache.' They occur on a nearly daily basis or every alternate day. Less severe forms resemble tension type headache. As the severity increases migrainous features become evident. The development of chronic headache is gradual. Initially there is occasional occurence and then the frequency increases. A recent American Migraine Prevalence and Prevention (AMPP) study has identified frequent migraine related nausea to be a marker for development of chronic migraine. There is an interesting report claiming to have an association of chronic migraine with vitamin D deficiency. However, it is not clear whether vitamin D deficiency is a cause or consequence of it.

Chronic headache is the most common type of headache seen in headache clinics. Approximately 1.5 to 2 percent of the population suffers from chronic migraine.

As the patients of chronic headache have near daily headache, their life is much disturbed. They are unable to do a regular job and their relationship with family; friends and colleagues are profoundly affected. They often develop depression.

Rebound Headache

People who overuse pain medication develop chronic migraine, this is called rebound or analgesic overuse headache.

'Amit used to have attacks of severe migraine three or four times a month. His doctor prescribed him an analgesic. With this, he got quick relief and now he need not miss his work. His performance improved and after six months he was promoted and was assigned greater responsibility. Following this, his migraine frequency as well as intensity increased. The analgesic was no longer that effective. Now he started to take two. This worked for few days, but he had to take analgesic more frequently. He realized that he was taking much more medicine. He consulted his doctor who prescribed an even stronger analgesic. This worked for few months, but again it became less effective. Now he was taking some or other analgesic daily and often more than once a day.'

Clearly Amit is suffering from rebound headache.

The most effective tool to determine whether one is rebounding is to keep a headache calendar. You should note the time and severity of migraine, the medicines taken, any other measure taken and what was the response. With the help of this calendar, you may know the

1. Pattern of worsening or increased frequency of headaches and the timing of its occurrence following discontinuation of medicines.
2. An increase in dosage of medicines being taken.
3. Preventive medicines or nonmedical treatment are no more effective.

In cases of rebound headaches, it is very important to change the treatment plan. Unless it is changed, the headache is unlikely to go away. Therefore, both the preventive medicines and the nondrug treatment plans have to be changed. Analgesics previously used, have to be stopped at all cost.

❑❑

8

CHAPTER

Migraine in Association with Other Non-Headache Illnesses

There are certain conditions and illnesses that are frequently accompanied by migraine. They are;

Psychological Disturbances

There is a complex relationship between psychological disorders and migraine. It is a fact that migraine is by no means an indication of depression or anxiety. But it has been that people with migraine are three times more prone to depression than those who do not have migraine. Likewise, anxiety (including panic) is much more common in migraine sufferers.

The other way is also true. Those who are depressed without migraine are more likely to develop it in the future than are people who are not depressed. Thus, this relationship is bidirectional. It may be assumed that perhaps there is a genetic predisposition to the development of migraine and depression in some people.

Therefore, it is very important to treat both migraine and the psychological disorders together.

Fibromyalgia

Fibromyalgia is a condition in which there is chronic, fluctuating, muscular type pain occurring in different parts of body like neck and back. Muscles are also tender (painful on touch). It is often associated with migraine and tension type headache. it is believed that in such patients, the pain system is hyper excitable.

Irritable Bowel Syndrome

In this benign condition the patient suffers from recurrent abdominal pain along with alternating diarrhea and constipation without any specific cause. It is commonly seen in migraine patients (and vice versa).

Restless Leg Syndrome

Restless leg syndrome is a condition in which the patient feels discomfort in legs (and occasionally the arms) in the evening and when attempting to sleep. There is an irresistible urge to move the leg making it impossible to stay in bed for very long and compelling them to get up and pace. The patient is unable to sleep unless he gets exhausted. Even in sleep there are periodic leg movements. Thus, the patient is devoid of a restful sleep.

Restless leg syndrome is more prevalent in people with migraine and fibromyalgia. The severity of restless leg syndrome is also documented to be on higher side in migraineurs compared with non-headache controls. Migraineurs suffering from restless leg syndrome report more premonitory symptoms. It is to be noted that antidepressants and antinauseants taken to treat migraine can exacerbate this condition. The patient should consult a doctor who can effectively manage this problem. Pramipexole is effective.

Raynaud's Phenomenon

It is a condition in which the hands become very painful on exposure to cold. It often co-exists with migraine. It can be exacerbated with certain headache medication.

❑❑

9

CHAPTER

Treatment of Migraine

Various treatment methods have been tried to control Migraine. It includes both pharmacological as well as non-pharmacological ones. The pharmacological method means treatment with use of medicines.

The treatment of migraine needs to control the acute attacks and to prevent further attacks.

Treatment of Acute Migraine

Acute migraine can be treated by both non-specific as well as specific medications. Among the non-specific drugs acetoaminophen 500 to 1000 mg per day is the weakest but safest medicine and it is preferable in children below 15 years age. It can be used alone or in combination with caffeine. Non-steroidal anti-inflammatory drugs (NSAID) like naproxen sodium 375 to 550 mg or ibuprofen 400 mg, diclofenac potassium

50 to 100 mg per day are effective, but often require an antinauseant like domperidone along with them.

Barbiturate containing medicines are quite often used for treating migraine, but it carries risk of medication-overuse headache. So they should be used only when other medication fails.

Opioids are to be generally avoided because they have tendency to cause addiction. Propoxyphene, butorphenol, meperidine, morphine, hydromorphone and oxycodone either alone or in combination with simple analgesic are very much effective and can be used in cases of severe but infrequent headaches. Opioids should not be used more than twice a week and it should be used only under strict guidance of a physician. Physicians often use it in short duration headaches like intractable menstrual migraine, since the headache improves when the menses is over.

Migraine patients often have disabling nausea and vomiting. Such patients need anti-nauseants which include certain neuroleptics (antipsychotics). Many of these drugs are effective for headache, even if there is no nausea. Metoclopramide 10 mg IV/IM, promethazine 10 to 30 mg orally or suppository, ondansetron 4 mg IV, chlorpromazine 12.5 to 25 mg IV, droperidol 0.625 to

2.5 mg IV/IM or prochlorperazine 10 mg can be given orally or intravenously or intramuscularly or by suppository. Many doctors prefer prochlorperazine intravenously or intramuscularly in their O.P.D or in emergency.

Droperidol is treatment of choice in cases of migraine lasting for more than three days (status migrainosus). ECG is to be monitored because droperidol may cause cardiac side-effects.

Corticosteroids like prednisone, hydrocortisone and dexamethasone are effective and may be used for short period of time, say about 7-10 days. It may be given orally or by injections. Prednisolone should be started with 20 mg TDS for two days then, 20 mg BD for two days then, 20 mg OD for two days then, 10 mg OD for two days then, 5 mg OD for two days and then stop. Similarly, dexamethasone should be started with 4 mg TDS on first day then 4 mg BD on second day then 4 mg OD on third day then 2 mg OD on fourth day then 1 mg OD on fifth day and then stop.

Ergotamine 1 to 2 mg orally and dihydroergotamine (DHE) 1 mg IM/IV/subcutaneous or 2 mg nasal spray are to be used, if analgesics fail. DHE is effective in most people. It can be given intranasally, intramuscularly, subcutaneously or intravenously. However, it should be used with caution in women of child bearing age group, cardiac, renal or liver failure patients. Ergotamine may induce abortion and cause birth defects.

Triptans are preferred treatment for most people with migraine. Though all triptans are effective, sumatriptan having been most extensively studied are used most commonly. About 80% migraineurs respond to subcutaneous sumatriptans, 60% respond with most oral triptans. However, the headache recurs, particularly in patients with long duration headache, which respond to a second dose of triptans. Triptans are contraindicated in heart patients.

Subcutaneous sumatriptans is the fastest and most effective. Sumatriptan or zolmitriptan nasal spray provides relief faster than oral triptans. Rizatriptan is perhaps the most effective oral formulation.

Amongst oral triptans—almotriptan 6.25 to 12.5 mg per day, eletriptan 20 to 40 mg per day, rizatriptan 5 to 10 mg per day, sumatriptan 25 to 100 mg per day and zolmitriptan 2.5 to 5 mg per day have the highest two-hour efficacy. They can provide relief in half to one hour. They are preferred where there is no problem of multiple recurrences and fast and effective relief is sought. Frovatriptan 2.5 mg per day and naratriptan 1 to 2.5 mg per day have lower efficacy, but have fewer side effects (as does almotriptan).

For patients who are prone to side effects almotriptan, frovatriptan and naratriptan are the best choices.

Here it is important to note that one triptan may be effective for a patient and a different triptan may be effective for another pateint. The earlier it is used, the better the response. Triptans can prevent cutaneous allodynia (nonpainful stimuli like combing producing pain).

At least two attacks with a new medicine should be tried, before concluding that it is ineffective. Migraine attacks should be treated as early as possible, particularly if the attacks are less than five per month. In more frequent attacks, it is better to identify the symptom which predicts that the headache will become severe.

Peripheral Anesthetic Procedures

Peripheral anesthetic procedures like nerve blocks have also been proved to be effective for bringing rapid headache relief with minimum adverse events. Greater occipital nerve blocks have given positive results in migraine patients specially with allodynia. Nerve blocks may be done on the following sites:

TABLE - 12

Nerve Block Procedures in Migraine	
Nerve Block Site	**Location**
Greater occipital	Medial to occipital artery, 1/3 of the distance between occipital protuberance and mastoid process
Lesser occipital	Lateral to occipital artery, 2/3 of the distance between occipital protuberance and mastoid process
Auriculotemporal	Anterior to the ear, superior to the posterior portion of the zygoma
Supratrochlear*	Above the medial border of the eyebrow
Supraorbital*	Above the eyebrow, about 2 cm lateral to supratrochlear nerve
* Supra orbital notch can be palpated easily and injection is to be given immediately above it in the eyebrow. Lidocaine (1% or 2% solution), longer-acting bupivacaine (0.25%-0.5% solution), or a combination of two agents, for the nerve block.	

Preventive Treatment

If the migraine attacks are frequent, preventive medications are needed to reduce attack frequency, duration or severity. It can be preemptive, short term, or long term.

When there is a known trigger like exercise or sexual activity, or a clear prodrome or aura, preemptive treatment is used. For example, a single dose of indomethacine 25 or 50 mg is given 1 to 2 hours prior to exercise to prevent exercise- induced migraine.

Short term prevention is used when the provoking factor is present for only a short period of time, like menstruation or ascent to high altitude. Treatment is taken for a short period when there is increased risk of headache. For example: using NSAIDs or Frovatriptan 2.5 mg daily for one week before the expected onset of menstruation for menstrual migraine.

Long-term prevention is recommended when there arc

- Very frequent attacks (more than two in a week).
- Disabling attacks even if attacks are infrequent i.e., only one or two attacks a month.
- Troublesome side effects or the drug is contraindicated or if the drug is ineffective.
- Overuse of acute medications.
- Risk of neurological consequences as in hemiplegic migraine.

During pregnancy, preventive medications should be avoided & Non pharmacological treatment should be the mainstay of migraine management.

The major medication groups for preventive treatment of migraine include beta-adrenergic blockers, antidepressants, calcium channel antagonists, nerve modulators and NSAIDs.

For prevention one of the drugs from the above-mentioned categories is chosen depending on side effect profile, patient profile and comorbid conditions. To start with, a low dose is given and increased slowly, unless side effects develop or maximum dose is reached. Usually, a low dose is sufficient for preventive purposes. It should be kept in mind that these medicines take about 2 to 4 weeks' time to start their action, and benefits may continue to increase over three months of therapy. So, a full trial of 2 to 6 months should be carried out. Premature withdrawal of medicines should not be done. Use of analgesics or ergot derivatives along with preventive medications should be minimized. Once the headaches are well controlled, the drugs should be withdrawn gradually.

Women of child bearing age should be on adequate contraception, and if pregnancy is being planned, preventive medicines should be withdrawn or it should be discussed with the patient and decision should be based after calculating the risk and benefits.

Preventive Medications

Beta Blockers

Beta blockers like propanolol 80 to 160 mg daily in two divided doses, Metoprolol 100 to 200 mg in two divided doses, nadolol 80 to 160 mg per day and timolol 10 to 30 mg per day are effective preventive medicines. However, beta blockers may produce behavioral side-effects, they are avoided in patients having psychiatric symptoms along with migraine. They are best suited for patients of migraine along with hypertension or angina. They are contraindicated in congestive heart failure, asthma, insulin-dependent diabetes and Raynaud's disease.

Anti-depressants

Antidepressants like tricyclics (TCAs), selective serotonin reuptake inhibitors (SSRIs), and selective serotonin and norepinephrine inhibitors (SNRIs) have been used successfully in prevention of migraine and tension type headache. Amongst these, amitriptyline (TCA) 30 to 50 mg per day, Nortriptyline (TCA) 30 to 50 mg per day and fluoxetine (SSRI) 20 to 40 mg per day have been extensively used and they have proved to be effective. Fluoxetine is very effective in chronic daily headache. Other SSRIs like sertraline 25 to 50 mg per day and escitalopram 10 mg per day are also effective. Side-effects like dryness of mouth, constipation and sedation are common with TCAs.

Calcium Channel Blockers

Calcium channel blockers like verapamil 160 to 240 mg per day in two or three divided doses and flunarazine 5 to 10 mg per day are commonly used, occasionally nifedipine is also used. They are quite effective and are especially helpful in hypertensive patients and in those patients where beta blockers are contraindicated as in asthma and Raynaud's disease. Verapamil is also effective in migrainous infarction or migraine with aura. Constipation and swelling of the legs may be some side effects.

Neuromodulating Drugs

Neuromodulating drugs (Anti-epileptic drugs) are the most accepted migraine preventing medicines. Of these, divalporex sodium and topirmate are proven to be most effective. The preventive dose is lesser than the anti-epileptic dose. Divalporex is effective at a dose of 500 to 1000 mg per day while topirmate is effective at 25 to 100 mg per day in two divided doses.

Neurotoxins

Neurotoxins like Botox have recently been found to be effective in preventing migraine. It weakens muscles by blocking the release of acetylcholine, a substance that transmits messages to the muscles. A clinical trial conducted at Jefferson Headache Center, Thomas Jefferson University Hospital, Philadelphia, Pennsylvania showed Botox to have reduced the migraine attacks significantly with no or minimal side effects.

Botox may be an effective and well-tolerated therapy for the prevention of migraine, tension-type headache and the headache of cervical dystonia. Its effect is long-lasting.

TABLE - 13

Medicine	*Starting Dose*	*Target Dose*	*Side effects*	*Contra indications*	*Beneficial for patients*
Beta Blockers					
Propanolol	20 to 40 mg BD ↑ by 40 mg every 1 or 2 weeks	80-160 mg per day in two divided doses	Fatigue, reduced exercise tolerance, bradycardia, hypotension, Broncho-spasm, sexual dys-function	Bronchial Asthma, uncontrolled heart failure, insulin dependent diabetes, patients having behavioral problem	Hypertensive patients Strongest evidence for efficacy
Nadolol	40 mg per day ↑ by 20 to 40 mg every 1 or 2 weeks	80-160 mg per day in two divided doses	same as propranolol	same as propranolol	same as propran-olol
Metopr-olol	50 mg BD	100-200 mg per day in two divided doses	same as propranolol	same as propranolol	same as propran-olol
Anti-depressants					
Tricyclic: Amitrip-tyline or Nortripty-line	10 mg per day (bed-time) ↑ by 10 mg every 1-2 weeks	25-50 mg per day	Sedation, drowsiness, urinary retention, weight gain, constipation, dryness of mouth, sexu-al dysfunc-tion	Cardiac patients, prostatic en-largement, Mania, uncontrolled glaucoma	patients having Insomnia, depres-sion, anxiety
Tetracy-clic: Mirtazap-ine	7.5 mg	15-30 mg at bed time	Sedation, weight gain, nausea, palpitation	Mania	Patients having Insomnia, depres-sion

SSRIs:					
Fluoxetine	10 mg	20-40 mg per day	Sleep problems, strange dreams, headache, dizziness, tremors, nausea	Mania	Patients having depression, anxiety
Sertralline	25 to 50 mg	50-100 mg per day			
Escitalo-pram	5 mg	10 mg per day			
SNRIs:					
Venlafax-ine	37.5 mg once daily for 1 week ↑ by 37.5 mg every 1-2 weeks	150 mg per day	dizziness, headache, anxiety, tremors, sleep prob-lems, strange dreams, nausea	Hyperten-sion, kidney failure	Patients having Anxiety
Calcium Channel Blockers					
Flunara-zine	5 mg per day at bed-time	10 mg per day at bed time	weight gain, depression, drowsi-ness, extra pyramidal symptoms	depression, parkinson's disease	Hypertension
Verapamil	40 mg BD for 1 week ↑ by 40-80 mg every 1-2 weeks	240 mg per day in two or three divided doses	Constipation, peripheral edema	Heart block, Bradycardia, hypotension, Congestive heart failure	Hypertension and in patients of ashthma or Raynaud's disease where beta blockers are contra indicated, migraine with prolonged aura

Neuro Modulating Drugs (Anti epileptics)					
Divalproex Sodium	250 mg per day for 1 week ↑ by 250 mg every 1-2 week	500-1500 mg per day in two divided doses	Nausea, vomiting, tremor, weight gain, loss of hair, increased hepatic enzymes, neural tube defects in neonates if used in pregnancy	Lever disease, bleeding disorders avoid in pregnancy	Strong evidence for efficacy in patients having seizure disorder, bipolar affective disorder
Topiramate	15 to 25 mg per day for 1-2 week then increase by 15-25 mg every 1-2 weeks	50-100 mg in two divided doses	Nausea, anorexia, renal calculi, paresthesia, acute glaucoma, dizziness, tremor, sedation, cognitive impairment, depression, weight loss, metabolic acidosis	Kidney failure, kidney stones, angle closure glaucoma avoid in pregnancy as there is small risk of encephalopathy when combined with valproate	

- Amitriptyline is the only drug that has been absolutely proven effective in migraine.
- Fluoxetine is of proven value in chronic daily headache and may work for migraine.
- Divalproex Sodium is the first neuro modulating drug proven effective in controlling migraine.
- Medicines usually take 2-4 weeks to act and the benefits continue to increase for over 3 months, therefore

medicines should not be prematurely stopped and should be continued for about 3-6 months.

Special Situations

Menstrual Migraine

NSAID like ibuprofen or naproxen and triptans may be used for miniprophylaxis. Some Gynecologists use oral contraceptives for three months continuously without any pill free day. This results in less menstruation and few headaches. The headache returns when the contraceptives are withdrawn.

Exercise Headache

For those who develop headache following exercise, they should warm up slowly. They may take a pain killer like indomethacin or ibuprofen or naproxen, before exercise and stay well-hydrated.

Non-Pharmacological Measures to Treat Migraine

A headache of migraine varies in intensity, frequency and duration amongst different patients as well as at different occasions in the same patient. There are several factors which do influence it. Many patients respond to various non-pharmacological measures, particularly when it is frequent.

A properly balanced life-style, including a healthy and balanced diet, regular sleep, regular exercise and a balanced out-look in different life situations; will almost always reduce the frequency and severity of headaches. The non-pharmacological measures may be categorized—dietary, physical and behavioral therapies.

Dietary Supplements

It includes vitamins, herbal or botanical preparations.

Vitamins

Various vitamin supplements have been found to be helpful in managing headaches. Riboflavin (vitamin B2), at a dose of 400 mg reduces headache frequency. Magnesium, if given intravenously, may treat acute attacks. Coenzyme Q, a nutritional supplement, if given at a dose of 150 mg twice a day is effective.

Vitamin B12 is also said to be of some help, as it is a nitric oxide scavenger, which is supposed to be involved in the production of headache. In cases of food and wine induced headache, histamine intolerance is believed to be causative factor of headache. Such patient should avoid such food and wine and a dose of 100 to 150 mg vitamin B6 (Pyridoxine) may be beneficial. There are some reports of long-term use of S- adenosylmethionine (SAM-e) to be effective in migraine treatment.

Though vitamins are helpful in managing migraine headaches, but too high doses can be potentially harmful. Therefore, a balanced diet containing all the necessary nutrients is essential.

Herbal Treatment

Herbs and other botanical produce have been used since ages and have been found to be useful in both acute pain and for a long-lasting effect. The most common therapies are:

- Inhalations using Melissa, peppermint, and chamomile.
- Massage with lavender, peppermint, anise, basil, and eucalyptus.
- Warm bath with eucalyptus, wintergreen and peppermint.
- Compresses of peppermint, ginger and marjoram, and vinegar.
- Combination of peppermint oil and eucalyptus oil, peppermint oil and ethanol.
- Other recommended treatments include warm salt packs, herbal footbaths, icy footbath, and cold sitz bath, cold and then hot baths, and tight headbands.

There are several others like butterbur, and feverfew. Amongst above mentioned, peppermint oil is supposed to be migraine-abortive.

Physical Treatments

Physical Therapy

Physical therapy in form of hot saline fomentation, massage, ultrasound or exercise is used to strengthen the neck muscle, improve mobility and to correct posture. For short term relief, hot saline fomentation, ultrasound and massage are effective and for long term relief exercise of neck muscles is very helpful. Many patients of headache feel tightness in neck and upper back. Loosening muscle spasms relieve migraine pain. Cold application with ice pack or vaso-coolant spray cools the skin and allows the therapist to stretch the tender muscles without pain. Cervical manipulation is also practiced and is helpful at times.

Acupressure and Shiatsu Massage

These are Asian methods of relieving pain. They are based on the principle that pain occurs as a result of blockage of energy flow, or Qi. In both methods this blocked energy is released by application of finger-pressure massage which targets the acupuncture meridians, 12 invisible energy channels throughout the body. The difference between the two methods is the intensity of finger pressure massage. In Shiatsu, it is less intense than Acupressure.

Acupuncture

Acupuncture is another Asian technique. It is based on the flow of the life energy force, Qi. Small needles are inserted into points along the meridians. It is said that acupuncture mobilizes serotonin and nor-epinephrine, which block pain transmission and produce endorphins, body's own natural pain-relieving chemicals.

There is difference of opinion about its usefulness in treating headaches. However as there is no evidence of harm, it can be tried as an additional measure.

Reflexology (Zone Therapy)

The principles of reflexology are similar to those of acupressure and shiatsu in that the areas and points on the hands, feet, head and ears correspond to other body areas. When the specific areas are massaged or pressure is given on it, it enhances the well-being of associated areas.

Qijong

Qijong is the skill of working with the 'life force' by using movement and meditation to reduce stress, blood pressure, and muscle tension.

Massage

Massage has been found to be effective in relieving pain. It helps relax muscles, release the tensions and other soft tissues, improve circulation, increase the uptake of oxygen, and stimulate the production of endorphins.

Yoga

Yoga is a traditional Indian ayurvedic practice. It means to unite or integrate. It is a way of life that trains the body, mind and emotions to unite the spirit. It increases the blood flow, releases tension, removes toxins, produce endorphins and regulate serotonin.

Apart from these other physical therapies are also in practice like chiropractic care and craniosacraltherapy. However, their results are non-conclusive and they also carry risk. Hydrotherapy is traditionally used as an adjunct to massage. It includes hot and cold packs, saunas, steam baths, and whirlpools.

Behavioral Therapies

Many patients of migraine who don't prefer drug treatment, or unable to tolerate it due to side effects, or when drug therapy is ineffective, or in cases of pregnancy, behavior therapy is used. It is often administered in small groups. It includes relaxation training, biofeedback therapy, and cognitive-behavioral or stress management training.

Relaxation Training

Relaxation training can be done by following methods:

- **Progressive muscle relaxation**: It is a method in which selected group of muscles throughout the body is tensed and relaxed alternatively.
- **Autogenic training:** It is a method of relaxation in which we promote deep relaxation by self-instruction of warmth and heaviness.
- **Meditation**: In this method, the mind is focused on a sound or mantra, to promote mental calm and relaxation.

As one learns to relax, he also develops greater control over his body. Relaxation training has been shown to be highly effective. One study showed that after 10 sessions of progressive muscle relaxation training, 96 % of migraineurs had a reduction in the frequency, duration, and severity of head pain.

Progressive muscle relaxation can be learnt with help of a video or auto tape. A series of toe-to-head muscle relaxation exercises are carried out. You start with your toes, contracting and relaxing individual muscles, and then work your way up, progressively covering all muscle groups. It is to be combined with deep breathing.

Relaxation can also be obtained by using visualization or guided imagery. Try to picture yourself in a relaxed state in your favorite place like a beautiful garden. Imagery or visualization causes same changes in the brain as if it were actually happening.

Meditation helps in reducing pain, high blood pressure, and heart rate. It also helps in reducing stress of daily life. Meditation is done by sitting in a relaxed position with closed eyes, and breathing deeply and slowly along with focusing on breath or some mantra. It is important to note that simply taking deep breathing brings relaxation.

Hypnotherapy – It has been approved by the American Medical Association in 1958 as a therapeutic technique. In this, the participant is highly receptive to suggestion in a state of focused concentration. It is effective in reducing the frequency and severity of pain in migraine and tension- type headache.

Biofeedback Training

Biofeedback is an established technique for prevention of migraine. it is more fruitful in children and young adults. It is mostly used in conjunction with relaxation training. In this technique, the person uses a physiological function to regulate the monitored response. For example, thermal (hand warming) feedback monitors skin temperature, whereby you can learn to control the temperature of your hands and feet. Electromyographic feedback monitors the electrical activity from the muscles of the scalp, neck, and sometimes the upper body.

Stress Management Therapy

Managing the stress is very essential to control headaches. Many patients develop headache as they are poor in handling their stress. They need to cope up with it. For this, it is important for them to look into their way of thinking and emotional components of their headache. The cause of stress needs to be identified and dealt with accordingly. If needed, life-style has to be changed. Stress management is used in conjunction with relaxation. Relaxation skills can be used throughout the day. Self-regulation skills can be practiced during pain free periods and may be utilized later on to abort an anticipated headache.

Psychotherapy

The headache sufferer usually gets distressed, feels helpless, frustrated, depressed and anxious. He needs psychological intervention. Psychotherapy can be done by counseling, cognitive therapy, behavioral therapy and support groups. They are helpful in dealing with the effects of disabling headaches.

Trance Cranial Magnetic Stimulation

This is a new invention for treatment of headache. The pain of migraine is believed to occur as a result of an electric storm. With the help of this new device, which is of the size and weight of a hair drier, two fleeting bursts of electricity is passed across the brain that short-circuit the electric storm in the brain, there by relieving the pain. Single shots make 39% persons pain free in two hours. After 24 hours 29% and after 48 hours 27% remain pain free.

Suggestions for Migraine Patients

- Before going to take the medical treatment try simple ways of handling pain, such as walking, neck massage, deep breathing, and relaxation technique.
- Change what you are doing. If you are cooking when headache starts, take a walk or read a book. Distraction is effective for many mild headaches.
- Have positive thinking. Replace negative thoughts with positive ones.
- Change your life-style.
- Have proper sleep with regular timing. Never deprive yourself from sleep.
- Take a balanced diet.
- Eat fresh food.
- Avoid food items which trigger your headache.
- Have regular timings of meals.

- ❖ Have a broad outlook towards life
- ❖ Avoid going out in the Sun, particularly in summer. If you have to go out, cover your head with a cloth/ towel. Use an umbrella.
- ❖ Avoid visiting places which are noisy or where there are glittering lights such as in marriage parties.
- ❖ Don't watch television/video from near distance or for a long period of time.
- ❖ Avoid using mobiles/computers for long duration (Say not more than 30-40 minutes at a stretch).
- ❖ Give rest to your eyes for 5-10 minutes, when doing any work where eye has to focus on a certain object for more than 30-40 minutes.

> A balanced outlook in life and meals with proper sleep and regularity in timings of meal and sleep are key points in managing headache.

❑❑

10

CHAPTER

Tension Type Headache

This is the most common headache. 80% of the people have experienced tension type headache at least once in life. So, it is the most familiar headache. Very little studies have been conducted on tension type headache despite it being the most common form of headache. Prevalence of tension type headache is much higher in Europe (80%) than in Asia and The United States (20% to 46%). The annual incidence was found to be 42.2 per 1000 person per year for frequent tension type headache in a Danish epidemiological follow up study with females three times more prone to develop it (male: female, 1:3). However, if all categories including infrequent, frequent and chronic subtypes of tension type headache is taken into account, females are only slightly more affected than males (male: female, 4:5). About 12% of episodic tension type headache convert to become chronic headache. About 2 percent of population suffer from chronic tension type of headache, about 10% have weekly headache and about 1/4 to 1/3 have several attacks in a month. About half the patients of chronic tension type headache achieve remission with treatment.

The headache may last for 30 minutes to seven days. The patient feels a dull, non-pulsating headache type of pain usually on both sides of head, it may be mild or moderate, as pressing or tightening over the head. The pain is often described as an external pain coming from outside. There is a feeling that a rope is tightened around the head. Some describe their pain as heaviness in head or feeling of a weight over their head and/or their shoulders. The muscles of the scalp, jaw and the neck may be tender. The headache is not associated with nausea or vomiting. Usually there is no relation with light or sound. The patient keeps doing his routine work. The headache is not aggravated by walking or climbing stairs. The stress of day-to-day life activities aggravate the tension type headache. Therefore, such headaches are worse in the evenings. Many people refer this headache as "just a headache." The pain may be episodic lasting for few hours, once or twice a year or may be continuous chronic constant pain lifelong. Many patients of tension type headache have migraine and medication overuse headache as co-morbidity.

The average age of onset of tension type headache is around 25-30 years which is higher than that of migraine.

Prevalence seems to peak between 30 and 40 years. There is only the slight decrease in prevalence of tension type headache with increasing age, whereas in migraine prevalence decrease is markedly observed after the 5th decade.

Though the tension type headache is episodic in nature, it may become chronic when its frequency rises to at least 15 days a month (daily or nearly daily) and it persists for more than three months.

"Arun was a 28 year-old sales representative. He used to have occasional headache in evening. The pain would be mild and he felt a tight band around his head. He was not disturbed by light or sound and he never had nausea or vomiting. He would take rest, massage his head and take a tablet of paracetamol and he would get relief with these measures."

Arun was suffering from tension type headache.

Tension type headaches are nondescript and usually non-disabling. However, considering the high frequency of tension type headache the overall disability caused by it on the population level is larger than that for migraine. Taken together (both tension type headache and migraine) headache has been ranked among 10th most disabling disorder. They often get relief with simple analgesics like acetaminophen and relaxation techniques.

TABLE - 14

Diagnostic criteria for the three subtypes of tension-type headache (ICHD-3beta) (Headache Classification subcommittee of the International Headache Society 2013)
2.1 [G44.2} Infrequent episodic tension-type headache A. At least 10 episodes occurring on <1 day per month on average (<12 days per year) and fulfilling criteria B-D B. Headache lasting from 30 minutes to 7 days C. Headache has at least two of the following characteristics: 1. Bilateral Location 2. Pressing/tightening (non-pulsating) quality 3. Mild or moderate intensity 4. Not aggravated by routine physical activity such as walking or climbing stairs D. Both of the following: 1. No nausea or vomiting (anorexia may occur) 2. No more than one of photophobia or phonophobia E. Not attributed to another disorder
2.2 [G44.2] Frequent episodic tension-type headache

As 2.1 Except for:

A. At least 10 episodes occurring on ≥1 but <15 days per month for at least 3 months (≥12 and <180 days per year) and fulfilling criteria B-D

2.3 [G44.2] Chronic tension-type headache

A. Headache occurring on ≥15 days per month on average for >3 month (≥180 days per year) and fulfilling Criteria B-D

B. Headache lasts hours or may be continuous

C. Headache has at least two of the following characteristics:

1. bilateral location
2. pressing/tightening (non-pulsating) quality
3. mild or moderate intensity
4. not aggravated by routine physical activity such as walking or climbing stairs

D. Both of the following:

1. no more than one of photophobia, phonophobia or mild nausea
2. neither moderate or severe nausea nor vomiting

E. Not attributed to another disorder

Causes of Tension Type Headache

There is no known cause of tension type headache. Some people with tension type headache have excessive contraction and ischemia of scalp and neck muscles and increased tenderness in these muscles. Therefore, it is also known as muscle contraction headache. Some studies have found high levels of anxiety, depression and suppressed anger in patients of tension type headache. However, there are no consistent findings in these patients in various psychological studies. It has also been seen that many patients do not have mood problem. So it is unclear whether tension lies in the muscle or in the mind.

It may be assumed that these patients are having stress in their life and they are not able to cope with it. They are not happy in their present circumstances. They find themselves entrapped with such problems, whose solutions seem to be apparently impossible. They find themselves in tight corners. They feel that there is no way out. Many times, their thinking is maladaptive. They may have misinterpreted certain events in their life and may be holding on to some wrong notions. Their outlook towards life may be negative. Not only this, they are so frustrated that they think that it will be futile to take any body's help. They hide their real problems. They do not want to discuss it. As a result, they keep suffocating themselves. They are always worried about one thing or other. They keep on thinking unnecessarily negative thoughts. So, at the end of the day, their brain gets exhausted and ultimately, they develop tension type headaches. It has been noted that depression increases the vulnerability to tension type headache which may further lead to depression.

Differential Diagnosis

A thorough history and proper physical examination is required to differentiate tension type headache from other types of headache. For this, patients should be asked to maintain a headache diary in which he should note all the details of headache, when and under what circumstances headache occurs, its duration, frequency, intensity as well as about factors triggering, aggravating or relieving headache, medication taken and its response.

- The most frequent differential diagnosis is Migraine.
- If the headache is progressive or there is a change in its pattern along with neurological sign and symptoms, intracranial space occupying lesion (Brain Tumor) is suspected.
- Over use of analgesics raises suspicion of medication over use headache.
- Visual symptoms, pulsating tinitus and increasing diffuse headache in an overweight person suggest idiopathic intracranial hypertension.

Treatment of Tension Type Headache

Episodic tension type headaches are treated with acute medications. More frequent or chronic headaches need preventive medication along with other non-pharmacological measures like counseling, stress management, relaxation therapy and biofeedback etc.

Medication

The treatment depends on severity of headache. In mild to moderate cases, simpler analgesics like Acetaminophen 500 to 1000 mg or Non-steroidal anti-inflammatory drugs (NSAIDs) like ibuprofen 200 to 400 mg, Naproxen Sodium 375 to 550 mg, Ketoprofen 25 to 50 mg and diclofenac potassium 50 to 100 mg have all been demonstrated to be effective in aborting tension type headache. At times, muscle relaxants are also used. The pain killers are taken alone or a combination with caffeine, sedatives or codeine may be used. If the headache is severe, the patient should take medicine as per advice of doctor who will prescribe medicines based on other associated symptoms, patient's clinical profile and previous response to treatment. He may prescribe a combination medicine or may consider a barbiturate like butalbital. Depending upon the frequency and severity of the headache, the doctor may start preventive medication. For this, the patient may be prescribed Tricyclic antidepressant like amitriptyline 10 to 75 mg, Nortriptyline 10 to 75 mg have proved to be effective. Even selective serotonin reuptake inhibitors (SSRI) like fluoxetine 20 mg or sertraline 50 to 100 mg or escitalopram 10 mg daily have also been found to be equally effective. Few studies have found even Mirtazepine 15 mg to be also effective. Their action in headache is completely different from their action against depression.

Anti-depressants like amitriptyline or nortiptyline should be started at low doses 10 mg per day and titrated by 10 mg weekly until good therapeutic effect or side effects are encountered. Common side effects are dryness of mouth, drowsiness, dizziness, constipation and weight gain. Usual dose is 30 to 70 mg given at bed time. The response may be observed in one to two weeks. At least 4 weeks trial should be given before switching on to other preventive medications. Preventive medication may be continued for 6 to 12 months.

Muscle relaxants are also used. Recently Botulinum toxin has been shown to be a primary treatment for chronic tension type headache.

Other Modes of Treatment

Physical Therapy

The patients of tension type headache associated with muscle spasm or tightness are fit patients for physical therapy. It consists of use of moist heat pads, ice packs, ultra sound and electrical stimulation; massage for short term pain relief, posture improvement by stretching, exercise and traction; and trigger point injections or occipital nerve block. The aim of physical therapy is to loosen muscle spasm, thereby improving mobility and relief from pain.

Psychological Factors

The psychological factors should be kept in mind. Often, patients suffer from various stresses, anxiety or depression. They may be causative factors or a consequence of headache. They need to be taken care of. The treatment includes counseling, stress management, relaxation therapy, biofeedback or medication.

Biofeedback

EMG biofeedback is a technique which enables people to control muscle tension by providing continuous information about the tension in one or more of the muscles. Such feedbacks may be auditory like clicks at variable rates or visual like bars of varying length. The sessions last for one hour. The treatment starts to work when people learn to either increase or decrease their head EMG activity.

Relaxation Training

Relaxation is very important for patients of tension type headache. The patients need to learn techniques of relaxation. There are two popular methods:

1. **Progressive muscle relaxation training:** In this, the patient learns to recognize tension and relax by sequentially tensing and then releasing various groups of muscles throughout the body. It can be

easily practiced at home daily on regular basis. For assistance, audio tapes are available in market.

2. **Autogenic training:** This is based on auto suggestion. The patient imagines and suggests himself that 'I am relaxing'. He concentrates on this. With regular practice he learns to relax and gets relief from headache.

Meditation

This is quite popular for producing mental calm and relaxation. One tries to focus his mind on a sound or silently repeated words (Mantra) during meditation. It has very good results. To meditate patients sits in a relaxed position, closes his eyes, takes deep and slow breathes, chants some mantras repeatedly and focuses on his breathe. This brings peace in your mind and the patient feels relaxed.

Cognitive Behavior Therapy

This is based on the assumption that people often have tension type headache due to maladaptive belief and thinking. They are trained to identify and correct their maladaptive thoughts. They are taught to look into the things in proper perspective. Consider it in totality and also look from the angle of other person's point of view. A broader vision helps in identifying the true problem and it also widens the scope of finding possible solutions.

Cognitive behavior interventions like stress management programs effectively reduce tension type headache. In people with a high level of daily stress, relaxation therapy or biofeedback need to be given along with cognitive behavior therapy. This gives excellent results and markedly reduces the dependency on drugs.

Apart from this balance diet, regular exercise and stretching, as well as adequate sleep, and maintaining regular sleep time are very important in controlling tension type headache.

❑❑

11

CHAPTER

Cluster Headache

The word cluster means 'a small close group'. Thus, cluster headache means multiple attacks of headache occurring in a small period of time. It is episodic in nature. There are cycles of daily, multiple, short duration headache lasting for 1-4 months and separated by remissions that last 6-24 months. The attacks often occur precisely the same time each day.

It is a rare condition. It occurs in 0.1% of the population. It is more common in males. Male-female ratio is 1:3.

This is one sided mostly around eyes, temple or near jaw, is very intense (excruciating), as if some hot poker is pierced into eye. It last from 15-90 minutes occurs 3-4 times in a day. The patient is usually awakened after one and half hour to two hours of sleep, nearly the same time each day. At times the eye is red and watering. There may be drooping of eyelid and swelling over face or eyelid. Nasal congestion and running nose may be present. Most of the times, the patient is very restless pacing to and fro and may even strike his head with wall and may injure himself. So it is also called "Suicidal Headache".

Most people have episodic cluster headache. If the attacks continue for more than one year it is called chronic cluster headache.

"Deepak, a young clerk of 25 years age, smoker, developed severe headache for several days while driving home after his duty was over at 5.00 p.m. The headaches always occurred over the right eye. It would last for one hour and were excruciating. His right eye appeared red and congested. Right eye would also appear swollen. His right nostril felt stuffy and there was watering from it. As he reached home, he would not sit still and paced rapidly. He felt irritated over trivial things. If his wife offered him a cup of tea, he would get angry. After one week he developed another attack (this was apart from the previous one) which would wake him up after two hours of sleep.

He consulted his doctor. After two months, he was relieved of the attacks. But they resumed the next year on the day they had started the year before. Based on his last year experience with these headaches, he was so terrified that, this time he consulted the doctor immediately."

Clearly Deepak was suffering from cluster headache as is evident from the facts of the typical symptoms, severity and precise regularity of the occurrence of the headaches. Deepak's cluster attacks are typical for age of onset, presence of smoking, male gender, number of attacks per day, and agitated behavior. (This is in contrast to the passive behavior of migraineurs).

Causes of Cluster Headache

Hypothalamus, a part of the brain is supposed to be involved in causing cluster headaches, as these attacks occur regularly each day at a particular time or at particular seasons. Hypothalamus is known to be the brain's clock. It is responsible for sleep and waking. Hypothalamus has been found to be activated during an attack in some neuroimaging studies using positron emission tomography. The pain is due to activation of trigeminal nerve which releases substances like CGRP which is responsible for sensation on most of the head and around the eye. Activation of the parasympathetic system a part of nervous system, releases a substance called VIP which leads to symptoms like running nose, sweating, swelling of eye lids. Another part of nervous system called sympathetic nervous system can be damaged due to swelling around the carotid artery. This may lead to droopy eye and small pupil on the cluster side.

Treatment of Cluster Headache

Cluster headache is a medical emergency. As the pain of cluster headache is very intense and there is a tendency to recur again and again people require rapid and effective treatment.

Maintenance Therapy

Preventive therapy should be started as early as possible, as the drugs take at least one to two weeks to act.

TABLE - 15

Preventive Medicines used in Cluster Headache

Medicine Name	Initial dosage	Maximal dosage	Remarks
Calcium channel blockers			
Verapamil	120 mg twice daily	240 to 480 mg twice daily	monitor ECG, (treatment of choice)
Anti-epileptics			
Divalproex Sodium	250 mg twice daily (extended release 500 mg once daily at bed time)	500 to 1000 mg twice daily	may cause hair fall, weight gain, increase liver enzymes
Gabapentin	900 mg daily	1800 mg daily	sedation (may be useful in refractory cases, Allodynia)

Topiramate	25 mg at bedtime	100 to 200 mg twice daily	Nausea, anorexia, renal calculi, paresthesia, acute glaucoma, dizziness, tremor, sedation, cognitive impairment, depression, weight loss, metabolic acidosis
Others			
Lithium Carbonate	300 mg twice daily	1200 mg in two divided doses	monitor serum levels (should not be more than 1.2 mEq/l)
Ergotamine	2 mg at bed time	3 mg at bed time	-
Dihydroer-gotamine	1 mg daily intravenous for refracto-ry cases	3 mg daily intravenous for refractory cases	antiemetic should be given prior to dihydro-ergotamine
Melatonin	9 mg at bed time	24 mg at bed time	

Drugs commonly used for preventive cluster therapy are verapamil, lithium carbonate, divalproex sodium and topiramate. Others like olanzapine and capsaicin cream—extracted from chili peppers are also possibly effective. In case of chronic cluster headache, if preventive drug therapy fails, surgical procedures like implanting brain stimulator in hypothalamus or occipital nerve stimulator can be tried. They are also said to be effective.

Transitional Treatment

As the preventive therapy takes time to act, transitional treatment is needed. For these, corticosteroids like prednisone, Medrol are used for short period of time. Prednisone should be started with 60-80 mg daily and tapered within 3 weeks. They should not be used for long term as they are not safe in the long term. Intravenous dihydroergotamine (1-3 mg) is effective in breaking an attack of intractable cluster headache. Occipital nerve block utilizing a local analgesic and corticosteroid on the side of headache is also effective.

Acute Therapy

Despite appropriate transitional or maintenance therapy, cluster headache may occur. Acute therapy shortens or aborts individual cluster attacks but does not prevent further attacks. Giving 100% oxygen for 10 minutes via a mask is safe and effective method of aborting a cluster attack. However oxygen treatment often just postpones the attack. Subcutaneous Sumatriptan as well as dihydroergotamine are very effective in aborting the attacks, but they should not be used more than twice a day. It may be noted that pain medicines, including opioids are ineffective in cluster headache.

TABLE - 16

Abortive treatment for Cluster Headache

Treatment	Efficacy	Remarks
100% oxygen (7-12 L/min) for 15-20 minutes	Relief in about 70% within 15 minutes	Very well tolerated
Sumatriptan 20 mg intranasally	Effective	May develop adverse events
Sumatriptan 6 mg subcutaneously	Highly effective	contra indicated in cardio-vascular diseases
Dihydroergotamine 1 mg intramuscularly or intravenously	Highly effective	contra indicated in cardio-vascular diseases

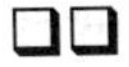

12 CHAPTER

Unusual Headaches

Apart from the usual primary headaches discussed in previous chapters, there are several unusual types of headache. Some of them are the following:

Paroxysmal headache: It is very rare. It is similar to a cluster headache except that they are much briefer and more frequent. They are well controlled by indomethacin.

Chronic daily headache: They last for more than 15 days in a month. The chronic tension type and chronic migraine has already been discussed in previous chapters. The rest include hemicrania continua & new daily persistent headache.

a. Hemicrania Continua

As the name suggests, it is a one sided continuous headache. It is of moderate severity which becomes severe at times. It is the least common chronic headache.

It is accompanied by nausea, sensitivity to light and sound, tearing, redness of eye and droopy eye lids. Thus it has features of both migraine and cluster headaches. Its cause is unknown. It may be continuous or remitting type. The remitting bout last from 1 to 6 months followed by a painless period of 2 weeks to 6 months. It invariably responds to indomethacin.

b. New Daily Persistent Headache

It starts suddenly and continues with constant unremitting pain. It is usually continuous, but there may be a painless period lasting for hours or days in some people. The patients do not have a history of worsening tension type headache or migraine. The cause is unknown. The Epstein Barr virus has been linkcd in some cases as it has been found around the time of flu-like illness. Stress has been found to be present in about 1 out of 8 cases. It is more common in women starting in their 20s. In men it commonly starts in 40s.

The patients have symptoms common to migraine like nausea, light and sound sensitivity, and pulsating headache. There may be aura like symptoms like zigzag lines and numbness in few cases. Stress, exertion, weather change, bright lights can aggravate the symptoms. MRI of the brain is almost always normal.

There is no specific treatment of the new daily persistent headache. Treatment is based upon symptoms. If symptoms resemble migraine it is treated like that and if symptoms are like tension type headache it is treated accordingly.

"Ice Pick" Headache

There are brief, sudden, severe jabs of pain resolving in few seconds (from 01-30 seconds only). It usually occurs as part of another headache disorder like migraine or cluster headache, but it may occur alone as well. It is usually infrequent few times a day, but may occur frequently throughout the day requiring treatment. It is almost never a long-lasting problem. There is no known cause. Though the pain is severe and very peculiar, people think it a serious problem, but experts believe that there is no need to investigate or look for a cause.

It is a very benign condition and does not warrant any treatment. The patient needs only reassurance. However, if the pain is frequent, indomethacin can be used, but pain reappears as soon as it is stopped.

Sexual Activity Headache

Headache occurring during sexual intercourse or masturbation is called 'coital headache'. Three types of coital headache have been identified. The most common type is a sudden explosive severe headache occurring at the time of orgasm. It lasts for hours and is very debilitating. It is very similar to the headache caused by rupture of an aneurysm which often is triggered by sexual intercourse. As headache due to rupture of aneurysm is life threatening, it is very important to rule it out when such pain appears for the first time. CT scan and spinal tap must be done as soon as possible to rule out bleeding aneurysm. Once bleeding aneurysm has been ruled out, the patients can be assured as most coital headaches are benign and generally resolve in few hours. It may or may not recur and sometimes occurs with each sexual activity. It can be prevented by taking indomethacin prior to intercourse. Migraine preventing drugs are sometimes effective and must be taken daily.

The second type of coital headache builds slowly and resembles as exercise induced migraine and is treated as migraine. The third type of coital headache is extremely rare and is like positional headache. Most pcoplc improvc spontaneously.

❑❑

13 CHAPTER

Secondary Headache

Headache occurring due to some other disorder is known as secondary headache. The common among them are discussed below:

Headache Due to Eye Problem

Many students visit headache experts for their problem of headache. Though they complain of feeling heaviness over their head, mostly over frontal area or over top of head, they also have problem of distant vision. However, they are not aware of this. Most of them have already taken painkillers before consultation. The eye problem is so common that in my out-patient clinic, amongst students ranging from 05 to 25 years who come for headache, about 30-40% of them are found to be having refractory error (difficulty seeing clearly objects placed at distant places known as Myopia).

As these students do not know that they have such problem they should be asked a simple question— do you have to copy notes from student sitting next to you? Do you have difficulty in reading the writings on the black-board?

When we are not able to see things clearly our muscles of the eye and surrounding area have to work harder to enable the things appear as clear as possible and this being a continuous process, they get exhausted and result in headache.

Eye check-up is must for young adults and children with headache.

Sinus Headache and Nasal Diseases

Sinus headache occurs due to infection or inflammation of sinuses (Sinuses are air filled spaces in skull). It is almost always preceded by infection of nasal structures. It is then called rhinosinusitis. Symptoms resemble migraine or tension type headache usually with common cold and fever along with pain in head and face, nasal congestion, running nose and pus discharge from nose. In acute cases, it lasts from one day to four weeks. Sub-acute cases last from 4 weeks to 12 weeks. If it persists for more than 12 weeks it is called chronic rhinosinusitis. Sometimes, acute episodes recur. If 4 or more episodes lasting for at least 7 days recur it is called recurrent acute rhinosinusitis.

Treatment is with antibiotics & decongestants along with steam inhalation.

Chronic rhinosinusitis is rarely a cause of headache. ICHD-II does not recognize chronic sinusitis as a cause of headache.

It is important to notice that many patients who think that they are having sinus headache, are actually suffering from migraine with weather changes acting as trigger.

In general, finding migraine among persons who think they have sinus headache is easy and it turns out to be almost everyone. It is unfortunate that the myth of sinus headache has prevented many people from being appropriately diagnosed and treated. Therefore, proper attention and care must be taken in properly diagnosing patients of headache who assume them to be suffering from sinus headache and then they should be accordingly& appropriately treated.

Deviated Nasal Septum

Rarely a Deviated Nasal Septum may cause one sided headache on the side the septum deviates. Such headache can be treated by placing a small piece of paper soaked in an anesthetic (lidocaine or Novocaine). Deviated nasal septum requires surgical straightening of the deviated septum.

Neck Problems

Problems of neck like cervical spondylitis, spasm of the neck muscles or other diseases of neck also produce headache which resembles migraine but it is present on only one side involving head and neck with pain increasing on neck movements. It never switches sides; occasionally, it can be bilateral. Headache may be present on awakening, or may begin after coming home from work, and may last for several hours. Later, headache may become continuous but diurnal variation in intensity may be there.

However, it must be remembered that all neck pains are not due to neck problems rather over half of migralneurs have neck pain during an attack. People with tension type headache also have pain in neck and head.

Those who keep their neck in a particular position for long period of time, for example those working on computers or type-writers, musicians, those talking on mobile for long duration with neck tilted on one side etc. develop headache as the pain arising due to stiffening of neck muscles is referred to head.

Developmental anomalies like fusion of head and upper cervical spine cause headache. Trauma to neck can cause headache. Rheumatoid arthritis of the upper cervical spine (cervical spondylitis) produces pain due to inflammation of synovial joints and stretching of the neck ligaments and nerves, Neck movements become painful. Pain killers and regular neck exercise do help.

Degenerative changes in bones and intervertebral discs (cervical spondylosis) start after 40 years of age and are very common. Not all cases lead to headache, as it mainly involves lower neck. Some of them do have headache typically in back of head, and often on one side.

Focal dystonia occurring in head and neck causes pain either due to continuous contraction of muscles or as a result of nerve irritation caused by muscular hyperactivity.

To make a diagnosis of headache caused by neck disorder, following specific features are required:

TABLE - 17

1. Pain occurring in neck and back of head, but pain may radiate to other parts of head or neck as well.
2. Pain may occur on one or both sides of head.
3. Patients, who have pain on one side, never switch to other side.
4. It must be possible to provoke the pain by particular neck movements or particular positions.
5. Neck movements should be restricted. There must be evidence of change in structure, contour or tone of neck muscle or increased sensitivity to pain on palpation.
6. An x-ray of the neck may show a straightened neck with loss of normal curvature.
7. CT or MRI may be required some times to rule out serious disorder like tumor.

Treatment

The treatment consists of both pharmacological as well as physical measures which are quite effective. A hot shower may give temporary relief. Mobilization, manipulation& massage gives comfort. Hot saline fomentation of neck provides relaxation. Regular neck exercise helps in relaxing neck muscles and thereby relieving pain. Cervical collar is also beneficial. At first it has to be worn day and night. However, if used too much it may lead to stiffness, weak muscle and pain. Patients are advised to avoid thick pillows. Rather a firm foam pad under the pillow or a Cervical pillow can be used.

The pharmacological treatment consists of pain killers, muscle relaxants, antidepressants, or sedatives. Occipital nerve block may be given.

Post Traumatic Headache

Post traumatic headache is one of the most controversial types of headaches. It is defined as headache following head trauma. While headache occurring within one week of an injury over head is recognized by all, there is a difference of opinion about the existence of chronic post traumatic headache. About 20% of acute post traumatic headache sufferers become chronic. This figure varies in different countries. It is high in countries like America where there is legal provision for compensation in cases of accidents, whereas in countries like Lithuania where there is no provision for compensation, it is low.

Cultural belief that long-term headache can result after injury actually causes chronic post traumatic symptoms has been suggested. It is seen in India, Japan, Europe, North America and many other countries.

Post traumatic headache is said to be chronic if it persists for more than three weeks. It is usually associated with sleep and mood disturbance. There may be problems of balance, concentration, memory and cognition. In real life situations this leads to lots of difficulties but formal testing is usually normal unless very sophisticated tests are performed.

The injury to head may cause symptoms as a result of concussion or stretching of axons and subsequent release of brain chemicals like NSE and S-100B into spaces surrounding the nerves. These same chemicals are also responsible for similar symptoms in insomnia.

It is important to note that even minor concussions in which, even if consciousness is not lost, there can be a permanent damage to brain functions.

In most people the headache and non-headache symptoms disappear, but become permanent in some. How this happens is not known. The head injury patients suffer lots of psychological stresses which add to their suffering.

There is no specific treatment for post traumatic headache patients. Treatment is symptomatic. Counseling and behavioral management helps in relieving some distress of patients. Many patients suffer from depression as well, which should be appropriately treated with antidepressants and cognitive behavior therapy.

Trigeminal Neuralgia and Atypical Facial Pain

Trigeminal Neuralgia

Trigeminal neuralgia is a condition in which there is a sudden burst of lancinating (severe darting or stabbing pain feeling like electrical shock) pain lasting from few seconds up to 2 minutes over one side of face and mouth. The pain occurs in attacks followed by a refractory period during which attacks cannot be triggered. There can be period of remission during which the pain disappears for months to years and then returns.

There are trigger zones in, discrete area of face or mouth which produces pain on being stimulated even by light touch. It is not necessary for the attacks to occur only on stimulation of these trigger zones. They may even occur spontaneously. People with trigeminal neuralgia often live in a perpetual fear of getting attacks of pain.

The cause of trigeminal neuralgia is supposed to be loss of the protective outer layer (myelin sheath) of the trigeminal nerve. The trigeminal nerve gets compressed by the artery or vein near its exit from the skull. It is called vascular compression. Diseases like multiple sclerosis cause the loss of this protective layer. Multiple sclerosis is to be a suspect in young patients if pain is present on both sides. Progressive symptoms and facial numbness may be more likely to suggest a secondary cause, such as neoplasm, brainstem infarct, Infection like herpes zoster, or syringobulbia. During acute attacks of Trigeminal neuralgia vasoactive intestinal peptide (VIP) appears elated and may enhance the effect of substance P, leading to pain.

Carbamazepine is the drug of choice. Other anti-convulsants may also be effective. If medication fails, surgery like micro vascular decompression is required which gives good results. About 80% get relief from pain following surgery.

Atypical Facial Pain

Patients who present with pain in facial region but do not fit the criteria of trigeminal neuralgia, are supposed to be suffering from atypical facial pain. There is no consensus amongst doctors about what is it exactly. The pain may be due to dysfunction of sensory nerves. Many patients present with severe, continuous pain in teeth (though there is no dental problem), with pain and numbness in one side of face on chewing. Some patients benefit with amitriptyline, an antidepressant.

Temporomandibular Disorder (TMD)

It is a disorder involving temporomandibular joint or muscles used for chewing. The joint-related problems may be due to inflammation or trauma, tumor, or congenital malformations. The muscular disorder may be due to spasm, muscle fatigue, regional muscle (myofascial) pain, infection or trauma to muscle.

TMD patients present with pain near jaw and the inability to open it. Treatment is with anti-inflammatory drugs, rest and physical therapy.

It is to be noted that if proper attention is not made in making a diagnosis, many times these patients are misdiagnosed and the patient keeps on changing doctors, like a Ping-Pong ball. It is important for headache sufferers to actively participate in diagnosis and treatment by providing detailed history and maintaining a headache calendar and discussing alternative modes of therapy. In complex cases, a multidisciplinary approach to therapy is advocated.

❑❑

14

CHAPTER

Management and Treatment of Headache

For proper management of headache, proper communication between the physician and the patient must be established. Both should communicate at an equal wave-length. The patient must tell his problem honestly and in detail, giving a comprehensive account of his symptoms, the previous treatment and its response. He should also be open in elaborating his stressors, about his life-style and the circumstances in which his headache starts or worsens, its timing etc. He must show interest in the treatment process. He should seek knowledge about his participation in complete treatment of his disease. To have knowledge about one's disease makes the treatment easier. Dependency on only drug therapy is not proper.

When a diagnosis is made, the patient must know it's meaning i.e., what is his disease, what is the possibility of his symptoms improving or worsening? When do these symptoms become alarming? When does he have to consult his doctor again? What can he do in this situation? Will a change in his life style help him control his headache? He must try to find out the stressors in his life which are making an impact on his symptoms.

Changes in the life-style may be small or big like doing yoga, walking, exercise particularly of the neck muscle, massage, deep breathing or relaxation by different techniques including biofeedback and progressive muscle relaxation. Even cycling and swimming may reduce intensity and frequency of headache. Major changes in life-style include change in home, or job. Change in environment or living condition may also bring a change in headache pattern. Changes in sleep habits like going to bed at proper time and using the bed for sleeping only; benefits the patient. Switching from a haphazard way of living to a relaxed way helps a lot in reducing the headache attacks.

It must be understood that for real benefit to occur, it will take few days. Real and regular relief is important than spontaneous relief. So in management of headache this point should be taken care of. For this purpose, the patient needs to be educated. The treating doctor must impart knowledge about the disease and the treatment process. Educating the patient is a skill and art. Every doctor should try to be proficient in this art. Regular practice and experience makes one perfect. It has been seen that imparting knowledge to patient in one setting is not of much help as patient is unable to understand and grasp it. So a regular dialogue between the patient and doctor should be continued in every session. The doctor should explain the things in the patient's language, keeping in mind patient's level of education, social background, and belief, so that he may be able to understand things easily.

For making a proper diagnosis and treatment a "Headache Calendar" is of much use. The patient must maintain this headache calendar which keeps details of headache accounts of the patients. When did the headache occur? For how long it stayed? What was the intensity? Which medicines benefited? Was there any side effects? etc. should be noted. Besides these, details about exercise, timings of lunch, dinner and sleep should also be recorded.

Real target should be set in cooperation with the doctor and the patient. It must be clear that it will take time for proper treatment. It is not possible to get relief in 05 minutes in severe cases. 1 out of 7 (around 15%)

get relief within 20-30 minutes of medication, whereas 60% get relief in 02 hours. If the pain is treated early, the results are better. No medicine works for ever. Few patients have successful treatment in 95% cases while others in only 80%. The patient also needs to know that every medicine has some side effects, which they have to tolerate. The doctor should prescribe the medicines as per the patient's profile.

Since primary headaches like tension-type headache, migraine and cluster headache don't have any definite cause; all the investigations are within normal limit. If the physician is assured about the diagnosis, unnecessary costly investigations like CT or MRI can be avoided. Here it is to be noted that many patients and their family members pressurize the doctors to have a CT or MRI be done, but it should be left to the doctor who is the best judge. This is very important for a country where most of the people are poor and such expensive investigations are not available everywhere. CT or MRI is required only when there is a suspicion of secondary headache like brain tumor etc., headache appearing for the first time after 45-50 years age, or if there is a sudden change in the nature of headache, it should be thoroughly investigated, as it may be of a serious nature.

Eye checkup is a must for children and young adults with headache as refractory error and convergence problem which is a common indication in this age group.

Primary headaches can be controlled, but cure is very difficult. It has been found that 50% patients get 50% relief in the intensity of pain. If intensity, frequency and duration of pain are reduced, it should be considered to be effective and beneficial treatment. Usually, 4 to 8 hours are required for control. It would be of value to note that the medicines take at least about 2 weeks' time to work. Therefore, treatment should not be changed before 2 weeks until there is some serious problem or side effects erupt. The drugs with property of sedation should be taken in night.

The triggers of headache need to be identified. Stress, excess or reduced sleep, change in weather, hormones etc. act as triggers. Some food items like ice-cream or red wine, caffeine withdrawal, chocolate, Cheese and other dairy products, citrus food like orange, lemon, grapefruit, pineapple and vegetable like onions, nut, beans as well as processed meat and fish and Chinese restaurant food which contain monosodium glutamate and food items made with sweeteners like Asparmate also act as trigger. As the patients of headache are sensitive to light and sound, they must take precaution. They should avoid going in sun, particularly in summers and that too at noon. The head should be covered with a cloth and an umbrella should be used. Similarly, they should avoid going in noisy places and where there are bright dazzling lights as in marriage parties. One must also try to avoid watching television from near distance and for long period of time. Mobile phones and computer should not be used for more that 30-40 minutes at a stretch.

It has also been observed that the chances of developing headache are enhanced, if one is unable to sleep properly, or keeps waking up the whole night. Such patients should avoid waking till late in night.

It has been observed that the patients of chronic headache usually take too much pain killers because the previous doses are no more effective now. Thus the dose and frequency of pain killers increase. This leads to rebound headache. In these patients the painkillers have to be withdrawn as rebound is an unhealthy behavior. They should be hospitalized. Intravenous dihydroregotamine regimen usually produces short term benefit.

Preventive treatment should be started if headaches occur more than once weekly. Once the patient attains and maintains adequate control for six months, it may be stopped. Preventive medicines like topiramate, or sodium valproate, amitriptyline or fluoxetine may be added which are quite effective. Onabotulinum toxin A is also effective. In some cases, nerve blocks are successful.

Avoidance of cigarette or bidi and regular exercise or yoga for 20 minutes is helpful. Neck exercises are important. Exercise reduces anxiety and tension in muscles, keeps the body energized and relieves it from tension. Bio feedback is also effective in some cases.

Trance cranial magnetic stimulation is a new and effective method. It gives relief very quickly, making patients pain free in just two hours in two-fifth cases.

Regular daily routine is very essential. A structured life-style with balance diet, balanced outlook, positive thinking, sleep and diet at regular and definite time, help in reducing headache. Good relationship with family and friends with proper and healthy communication, easy going and tension free life-style are all very helpful in managing headache.

Thus, a comprehensive approach is needed for managing headache.

Here I recollect what my revered teacher professor A.K. Agarwal used to say “To be a successful doctor don’t treat the disease, treat the person as a whole,” and that stands true for successful management of headache also.

❑❑